Plz return d
Lou Farley
410 Grand Ave., Ste. 307
Laramie, WY 82070

AT LAST . . .
EVERYTHING YOU NEED TO KNOW
ABOUT ST. JOHN'S WORT—
THE LATEST MEDICAL NEWS,
GUIDELINES FOR TREATING DEPRESSION,
PLUS INSTRUCTIONS FOR OTHER CONDITIONS!
BE INFORMED ABOUT . . .

- Side effects, including an important caution for fair-complexioned users
- Full instructions for growing the herb in a garden of your own
- The one word you must find on a St. John's wort product's label . . . or else don't buy it
- A healing *footbath* that not only soothes aching feet, but can help fight an oncoming cold
- Improved sleep patterns in as little as seven days
- Weight loss help, including an end to bingeing and overeating
- Higher energy levels in two weeks
- An analgesic herbal bath for menstrual and menopausal discomforts
- The newest findings on antiviral action against influenza A and B, herpes simplex, Epstein-Barr, vesicul equine infectious anemia, Hepatitis C, and

AND MUCH MORE

QUANTITY SALES

Most Dell books are available at special quantity discounts when purchased in bulk by corporations, organizations, or groups. Special imprints, messages, and excerpts can be produced to meet your needs. For more information, write to: Dell Publishing, 1540 Broadway, New York, NY 10036. Attention: Director, Special Markets.

INDIVIDUAL SALES

Are there any Dell books you want but cannot find in your local stores? If so, you can order them directly from us. You can get any Dell book currently in print. For a complete up-to-date listing of our books and information on how to order, write to: Dell Readers Service, Box DR, 1540 Broadway, New York, NY 10036.

ST. JOHN'S WORT

THE MIRACLE MEDICINE

❖

Alan H. Pressman, D.C., Ph.D., C.C.N.

WITH NANCY BURKE

PRODUCED BY
THE PHILIP LIEF GROUP, INC.

A DELL BOOK

Published by
Dell Publishing
a division of
Bantam Doubleday Dell Publishing Group, Inc.
1540 Broadway
New York, New York 10036

If you purchased this book without a cover you should be aware that this book is stolen property. It was reported as "unsold and destroyed" to the publisher and neither the author nor the publisher has received any payment for this "stripped book."

Neither this nor any other book should be used as a substitute for professional medical care or treatment. It is advisable to seek the guidance of a physician or other qualified health practitioner before implementing any of the ideas or procedures suggested in this book in regards to your health. This book was written to provide selected information to the public concerning the herbal remedy, St. John's wort. Research of this herb is ongoing and subject to interpretation. Although we have made all reasonable efforts to include the most up-to-date and accurate information in this book, there is no guarantee that what we know about this complex herbal remedy won't change with time. The reader should bear in mind that this book is not intended to take the place of medical advice from a trained medical professional. Readers are advised to consult a physician or other qualified health professional regarding treatment of all of their health problems. Neither the publisher, the producer, nor the authors take any responsibility for any possible consequences from any treatment, action, or application of medicine or preparation by any person reading or following the information in this book. All the names herein have been changed to protect their identity.

Copyright © 1998 by The Philip Lief Group, Inc.

All rights reserved. No part of this book may be reproduced or transmitted in any form or by any means, electronic or mechanical, including photocopying, recording, or by any information storage and retrieval system, without the written permission of the Publisher, except where permitted by law.

The trademark Dell® is registered in the U.S. Patent and Trademark Office.

ISBN: 0-440-22605-8

Printed in the United States of America

Published simultaneously in Canada

July 1998

WCD   10   9   8   7   6   5   4   3   2   1

To my son, Corey,
and my daughter, Meghan,
because they are my life

Contents

Introduction

In the past eighteen months, more than half a dozen books have been published about St. John's wort *(Hypericum perforatum)*, a centuries-old plant herb whose medicinal uses have long been esteemed by traditional herbalists. This plethora of books—most of which focus on the antidepressant benefits of St. John's wort, but hint at its other healing properties—heralded an unprecedented and widespread interest in a plant that many had previously viewed only as a nuisance weed.

Soon news of a "wonder drug" from the plant kingdom—one that could treat a range of illnesses as varied as depression, AIDS, tuberculosis, influenza, as well as bedwetting—spread as prolifically as the wild-growing weed itself does.

The seemingly miraculous benefits of St. John's wort have been touted on prime time television shows and in newspapers, magazines, and medical journals. If you take a casual stroll through the Internet and visit any of the natural health and herbal medicine websites, you will see an extraordinary trend in full sway: scores of people using St. John's wort for an astonishing variety of reasons and conditions. Then there are the many more people requesting information about how they can begin using St. John's wort. Health food stores are having a difficult time keeping this relatively unknown herb in stock, and it even has its own website.

It would seem that modern medicine and the public-at-large are just discovering the natural healing benefits of St.

John's wort, just as they have "discovered" ginger, echinacea, and ginkgo biloba in the last five years.

But in fact, St. John's wort has been the subject of intense scientific research for more than thirty years, and European doctors have prescribed it for depression for at least twenty years. And while it may seem that the skeptical American medical establishment is only now taking a serious interest in St. John's wort, partly in response to incredible public interest in the herb, this is only partly true. Indeed, it was an American team of scientists, working in collaboration with Israeli researchers, who discovered the potentially potent anti-AIDS properties of St. John's wort ten years ago. Now the Food and Drug Administration (FDA) has sponsored a multicenter research project that will study the effectiveness of St. John's wort in treating depressed patients at hospitals and clinics throughout the United States.

The results of the FDA study are a few years down the road and, for now, St. John's wort remains an unregulated plant "medicine" that is readily available over the counter in health food stores, herbal emporiums, supermarket chains, and larger pharmacies. Growing numbers of people, bolstered by the information they've gleaned from books, newspapers, and the Internet about the effectiveness and safety of St. John's wort, are using the herb on their own, primarily to treat depression, but also for other illnesses and conditions.

We have written this book precisely for those people. Though much of the scientific evidence does indeed point to the fact that St. John's wort is remarkably safe and effective in treating many conditions, especially depression, it is potent medicine nevertheless and should always be viewed as such. In fact, many of its therapeutic properties are still under investigation and will be for quite some time, including its long-range side effects, interactions with other drugs or other medical conditions, and possible toxicity when used during pregnancy or in young children.

With this book, we hope to dispel some of the "bandwagon" mentality surrounding the use of St. John's wort and help you make an informed and measured decision about whether it is the right medicine for you. And because throughout the book we recommend you take St. John's wort only in partnership with a qualified medical practitioner, this book is also for your conventional or alternative practitioner. Here you both will find the latest medical news about St. John's wort and, for the first time, suggested guidelines for using the herb to treat conditions other than depression.

Part I of the book begins with a look at the long history of St. John's wort and both its fabled and its factual uses through the centuries. Then we provide an in-depth description of the major chemical compounds found throughout the plant, detailing their specific therapeutic properties based on current research. Following that, we discuss whether St. John's wort is right for everyone, and we describe its possible side effects as well as situations where it shouldn't be used at all. Finally, we discuss how to buy, take, and even grow high-quality St. John's wort.

Part II of the book focuses on using St. John's wort to treat various illnesses and conditions. Here, the most indepth discussions about using St. John's wort focus on its benefits in treating depression—by far its most popular and well-studied application—and on its potential for effectively treating some of the symptoms and problems of premenstrual syndrome (PMS), menstruation, and menopause. We also look at some of the newly discovered therapeutic uses of St. John's wort and suggest ways you might use the herb to treat insomnia, fight viruses, strengthen

immunity, and achieve weight loss. Throughout this section we also make suggestions about using St. John's wort
with other herbs in medicinal teas.

Finally, we take a brief look at the possible directions
that future research and use of St. John's wort will take.
We conclude the book with a helpful listing of herbal suppliers and information resources.

Our approach throughout the book is measured, cautionary, but always enthusiastically supportive. As such,
perhaps we are not unlike the biblical prophet for whom
St. John's wort was named. We, too, are voices crying in a
new wilderness, where alternative and conventional medicine are having a profound but still tentative meeting of
the minds.

The overwhelming body of research about St. John's
wort strongly suggests that it may have more therapeutic
potential than any other medicinal herb currently under
study. This is great news. Furthermore, it does appear to
be remarkably safe for most people in most situations.
This is also good news. Nevertheless, misinformation still
abounds about this extraordinary herb. And far too many
people are taking it, particularly for depression, without
consulting with a medical practitioner.

Our hope is that this book will both dispel some of the
misinformation surrounding St. John's wort and encourage
people to try this remarkable herb under the guidance of a
practitioner. We wish you luck and good healing.

PART I

❖

An Introduction to
St. John's Wort

CHAPTER 1

❖

The Story of St. John's Wort

Its virtue cannot be described; how great it is and how great are its uses. And in all formulas there is no medicament that is so good and without detriment, without hazard, as the healer St. Johnswort . . . its virtue shames all formulas and doctors, they may cry as they may.
—PARACELSUS, GERMAN-SWISS
ALCHEMIST AND PHYSICIAN, 1493–1541

Clinical trials suggest that hypericum [St. John's wort] might become an important tool for the management of depressive disorders, especially in primary care settings.
—BRITISH MEDICAL JOURNAL, 1996

ST. JOHN'S WORT: MAGIC AND MYTH MEET MEDICINE

In late June, when the summer solstice draws near and the sun is at its apex in the northern sky, a perennial plant with bright yellow blossoms blooms in abundance along superhighways and country roads, in fields and meadows, woods and gardens. Its petals and leaves, covered with small black translucent dots, produce a deep red oil when they are bruised or rubbed. As one legend has it, in the early days of Christianity this crimson-colored oil was believed to symbolize the spilled blood of the first-century martyr St. John the Baptist, whose birthday is celebrated on June 24, near the time of the summer solstice. And so the plant came to be known as St. John's wort (*wort* being the Middle English word for "plant").

It is called many other names as well: *qian ceng lou* in China, where it has been listed in that country's esteemed herbal pharmacopeia for thousands of years; *Johanniskraut* in Germany, where it is prescribed twenty-five times more often for depression than the conventional and far more costly antidepressant Prozac; and *zwieroboij* in Russia, where Ukrainian scientists were studying its antiviral and antibiotic properties nearly thirty years ago. In the American West, where it is considered a nuisance weed, St. John's wort is known both as *Klamath weed*, after the great California river along whose banks it grows, and as *goat weed*, because of that animal's keen fondness for grazing on it.

Weed or not, from antiquity through modern times St. John's wort has been put to startlingly diverse uses, from healing wounds to fighting demons, from relieving pain to curing insanity. Along the way, ancient healers, shamans, and practitioners of folk medicine have honored the plant's many healing properties by variously calling it the Devil's Scourge, Grace of God, Penny John, Witch's Herb, Tutsan, and God's Wonder.

Present-day naturopaths, herbalists, and homeopaths— together with the ever-growing number of people who consult them—know this common weed simply as St. John's wort. And they have long touted its many extraordinary healing properties.

Now conventional doctors and research scientists are discovering—and, more important, confirming—what alternative medical practitioners knew all along: a freely growing weed that can be found virtually worldwide may be the key to treating a wide range of physical and emotional conditions effectively, safely, naturally, and economically.

Even as this book goes to press, medical researchers around the globe are studying the therapeutic benefits of St.

John's wort for AIDS, cancer, hepatitis, tuberculosis, cardio-vascular disease, insomnia, attention deficit disorder (ADD), and obesity. And based on Germany's well-documented success in treating depression with St. John's wort, the U.S. Food and Drug Administration (the notoriously conservative FDA) has recently announced it will sponsor a multi-million-dollar research study of the plant's antidepressant properties under the auspices of the National Institutes of Health and the Office of Alternative Medicine.

Clearly St. John's wort has traveled an impressive road from its folk origins in antiquity—where its use was shrouded in both fact and fantasy—to its newly venerated status as a "miracle" drug for the modern world—where it may well provide the critical and ultimate nexus between alternative medicine and conventional medicine. St. John's wort is now the most famous member of a mighty arsenal of medicinal plants recently "rediscovered" by mainstream science, but long esteemed by traditional herbal medicine.

HERBAL MEDICINE AND THE SCIENCE OF "LIKE TREATS LIKE"

One of the earliest references to St. John's wort comes from the first-century Greek botanist Pedanios Dioscorides, physician to the Roman emperor Nero and author of one of the first Western *materia medica* (a compendium of therapeutic plants). Dioscorides described St. John's wort as a superior vulnerary (wound healer) and diuretic, and as a pain reliever especially effective for neuralgic conditions such as sciatica. His Greek and Roman contemporaries, Galen and Pliny, echoed the Greek botanist's high praise for the plant, and other physicians of the time remarked that St. John's wort also was an excellent emmenagogue (a plant herb that stimulates and regulates menstrual flow), as well as a fever reducer.

In fact, most of the first recorded references to St. John's wort come from herbal scholars and physicians of the Greek and Roman empires, where the plant was known by its Greek name *Hypereikon*. Like most celebrated herbs whose healing properties have been esteemed through the ages, the benefits of St. John's wort—both medicinal and mythical—were no doubt well known, passed down orally by generations of indigenous herbal healers before recorded history began.

Knowledge about the effectiveness of St. John's wort in treating wounds and inflammations, for example, certainly would have been long-standing. Most early healers followed the ancient folk belief that the physical characteristics of a medicinal plant were related to the conditions it treated most effectively. The blood-like oil extracted from the flowers and leaves of St. John's wort suggested to the ancients that the plant would be effective in treating wounds, burns, and inflamed infections—as indeed it was.

This therapeutic principle of "like treating like," or *similia similibus curentur*, has long been promoted by folk healers and certain physicians and scientists. Hippocrates, the father of medicine, wrote about it in the fifth century B.C., theorizing that there were two types of medical treatment: the healing by opposites and the healing by "similars." Through subsequent centuries the principle of "similars" was elaborated on extensively (and sometimes speciously) and extended to most herbs used in treating illnesses.

By the Middle Ages this principle was formalized as the controversial "Doctrine of Signatures," the belief that God left "signatures" or clues in the plants he created about how to use them medicinally. Thus a plant with spotted leaves was believed useful in treating lung ailments, while a plant with kidney-shaped leaves was believed useful for treating illnesses of the urinary tract.

In the sixteenth century, the radical but brilliant Swiss-German physician, Paracelsus, often viewed as the "father of chemistry," became the most vocal advocate of the principle of "like treating like." To that end, he championed the systematic study of plant herbs from a chemical perspective, with special emphasis on the use of single herbs in precise dosages. An early proponent of the germ theory of medicine, Paracelsus proposed the idea that small doses of the same "poison" that caused an illness could also cure the illness. But he was roundly criticized for that belief, and his theories lay dormant for two hundred years.

By the late eighteenth century, however, during the European Age of Enlightenment—a time when both rational thought *and* political and intellectual freedom were encouraged—the principle of "like treating like" regained popularity and became the basis of homeopathy, an alternative healing method that relies heavily on natural herbs.

Herbal medicine moved out of the realm of simply folk medicine and was widely practiced among all classes in Europe for the next hundred years. But by the late nineteenth century, conventional or "allopathic" medicine, with its almost exclusive emphasis on synthetic drugs and surgery, took prominence as the preferred healing method of the upper and middle classes. Herbal medicine was now regularly debunked as superstitious nonsense by the more "scientific" medical establishment, and its practice fell out of favor with all but the working and peasant classes. They had successfully used herbs for centuries and couldn't afford the new "medicine" anyway.

Some debunking of the old methods was necessary, of course. For example, most plants with spotted leaves were thoroughly *ineffective* in treating lung ailments, contrary to what the ancient practitioners of the Doctrine of

Signatures had believed. Other plants were downright poisonous when they weren't simply ineffectual. But many other therapeutic plants were powerful healing aids. They did exactly what they were supposed to do, and they did it more effectively and less expensively than the newer drugs, with far fewer side effects.

St. John's wort was one of these potent healing plants, and it simply wouldn't go to ground when conventional medicine took prominence. Furthermore, as we shall see, St. John's wort would maintain its esteemed standing through centuries of fabled and fanciful usage only to go on and prove itself on both sides of the Atlantic—as an excellent treatment for wounds and infections—in the most pragmatic of laboratories, the battlefield. And it was there, no doubt, while investigating St. John's wort as a wound healer, that traditional practitioners soon discovered its many other extraordinary properties.

A PLANT BY ANY OTHER NAME . . .

The official botanical name for St. John's wort is *Hypericum perforatum (H. perforatum)*, though it is usually referred to simply by its genus name, hypericum (something we do throughout much of this book). The Latin species' name, *perforatum*, is a reference to the tiny black dots found on the plant's flowers and leaves. To the naked eye these dots look like holes or perforations, but in fact they are small glands from which the plant's red-colored oil is extracted.

As for the plant's genus name, scholars have offered several explanations about the derivations both of *Hypereikon*, the plant's original name, and of *Hypericum*, the name by which we know it today. Some scholars believe *Hypereikon* is simply derived from the Greek words *hypo* (under) and *ereike* (heath or heather), which translates to "under the heath" or "under the heather," perhaps an ancient reference to where the plant could be found.

Other scholars believe the better-known *Hypericum* comes from the Greek *hyper* (over) and *eikon* (icon or apparition) and means "over an apparition," a reference to the folk belief that St. John's wort possessed a protective power over evil and could drive away demons. This belief persisted from early antiquity right through the Middle Ages. In the sixth century, as one legend has it, the plant was further immortalized by the beloved Celtic saint, Columba, a devotee of St. John the Baptist. St. Columba, who established monasteries throughout Ireland and Scotland, was said to carry a sprig of St. John's wort with him wherever he traveled in honor of the martyred saint. But he might also have carried St. John's wort for spiritual protection during his long and dangerous travels as a missionary to the Celtic tribes.

By medieval times, St. John's wort was part and parcel of many summer solstice rituals. On the eve of St. John's Day, for instance, it was common practice to hang wreaths made from the plant's leaves and flowers on the doors of homes and churches as protection against witches and other evil spirits. People also placed sprigs of the plant under their pillows on St. John's Eve, in the belief that St. John himself would appear to them in a dream, give them his blessing, and prevent them from dying during the year that followed. And the dried leaves of the plant were considered protective talismans, frequently used as bookmarks in Bibles and prayer books.

It is easy to understand how some of the ancient superstitions that surround St. John's wort arose. The plant blooms wildly and abundantly near the date of the summer solstice, an important planting time that is historically rich in pagan, native, and early religious rituals. Offerings were made to the ancient gods and goddesses of the Sun and Earth for a fertile growing season; prayers were proffered to Western saints for bountiful harvests in the fall.

This is also the time that marks the celebration of the birthday of St. John the Baptist, himself a wild and iconoclastic early saint who lived as a desert hermit, surviving only on locusts and honey—and, as some legends would have it, also on the plants the locusts were drawn to, namely, St. John's wort. John the Baptist was martyred as a young man in particularly gruesome fashion, and his decapitated head was served up on a platter to the evil dancing girl Salome.

This latter piece of biblical history, together with the fact that the plant's oils leave blood-like stains on the fingers and hands of those who pick it, certainly gave rise to some of the magical and sinister connotations associated with St. John's wort.

ST. JOHN'S WORT: THE MEDICINE IN THE MYTH

On the other hand, the ancient belief that St. John's wort offered protection against evil spirits and bad luck may have risen in part from its early use by traditional healers as a treatment for what was called "melancholia" or troubled spirits. Today we call these conditions depression or anxiety; indeed, St. John's wort has attracted the most attention in recent years for its antidepressant properties.

In antiquity, however, the plant's effectiveness in treating mental and emotional illness was no doubt inadvertently discovered—though perhaps little understood—as a side effect of one of its more common uses. Ancient healers and herbalists who routinely treated people's wounds and infections with St. John's wort most likely noted that the plant also had a calming or sedating effect, particularly in its pure oil form, when it was applied directly to (and absorbed by) the skin, and in its liquid form (made from steaming the plant's leaves and flowers—what is called an "infusion" in traditional herbal medicine), which was taken internally.

Certainly by the Middle Ages both therapeutic uses of St. John's wort were common practice. Knights of the Order of St. John of Jerusalem regularly used poultices made from the crushed flowers and leaves of St. John's wort to stop bleeding and treat injuries on the battlefields of the Crusades throughout the eleventh, twelfth, and thirteenth centuries. During the same period, those suffering from mania, or believed to be possessed by demons, were frequently treated with infusions of the plant or made to inhale its slightly bitter, vinegar-like odor.

———————————— ❖ ————————————

Kathy's Story: Helping Her Son's ADD

The newest investigations for uses of St. John's wort include therapeutic treatments for obsessive-compulsive disorders (OCDs) and attention deficit disorders (ADDs), particularly among young adolescents. While there is no hard-core clinical research as yet on these particular therapeutic applications of St. John's wort, many parents have used the herb, under the guidance of a medical practitioner, to help relieve their children's OCD and ADD symptoms and to avoid the use of heavy prescription medications with their accompanying side effects.

Kathy, a forty-two-year-old stay-at-home mom, has had great success using St. John's wort to treat her thirteen-year-old son's OCD: "Our experience treating our son with St. John's wort has been really encouraging. We

had tried both prescription antidepressants and psychotherapy, but neither was helping much. The drugs did
little to relieve his symptoms, and he had some terrible
side effects—angry and aggressive behavior at home
and in school and a lot of trouble concentrating on his
schoolwork. A friend of ours who's been into holistic
medicine for years told us about St. John's wort, and after reading some of the literature and talking to our
son's therapist, we started giving him St. John's wort—
six hundred milligrams a day.

"Our son's been on St. John's wort for almost four
months now, and there's been a dramatic decrease in
his OCD symptoms—they're more manageable than
they've been in years! Plus he has fewer mood swings
and flare-ups, and there are none of the side effects
he had with some of the prescription antidepressants.
His whole attitude has improved and his mood is more
upbeat.

"I've shared this in the hope that other parents who
are looking for an alternative to prescription drugs for
their children will be encouraged and at least talk to
their doctors about trying St. John's wort."

❖

ST. JOHN'S WORT:
MUCH MORE THAN A WOUND HEALER

Other uses for St. John's wort were soon discovered by established herbal medical practitioners, though they had
long been known in folk medicine. The plant's somewhat
bitter, balsamic odor and taste suggested that the herb was
also an astringent (herbs traditionally used as diuretics and

to treat urinary tract infections). In the late sixteenth century, the great English herbalist John Gerard noted that St. John's wort "provoketh urine, and is right good against stone in the bladder." Gerard also noted that St. John's wort was an excellent healer of wounds, burns, and insect bites. In 1618, St. John's wort was one of the medicinal plants listed in the first *Pharmacopoeia Londonensis*.

In folk medicine, especially that practiced by women shamans and herbalists, St. John's wort also had a long-standing use as a "female tonic" and was regularly prescribed to stimulate and regulate menstruation, relieve muscle spasms, and boost the spirits. It was also used to treat kidney ailments, especially enuresis (bed-wetting), to expel worms, and to relieve nerve pain. Gerard's Italian contemporary Mattioli confirmed the plant's effectiveness as an emmenagogue and also noted that St. John's wort was an excellent treatment for malaria—an early reference to the plant's antibacterial properties, which are now the subject of much research.

American colonists who immigrated from England, France, and Germany brought St. John's wort to the northeastern United States, and from there it spread throughout much of the country as colonists moved south and west. During the country's Revolutionary period, St. John's wort was widely known for its wound-healing properties, and no less than Benjamin Franklin noted that "lacerated wounds of parts rich in nerves yield nicely to this drug." One hundred years later, when American herbalism flourished during the Eclectic period, esteemed herbalists John King and Finley Ellingwood noted that the use of St. John's wort had now extended way beyond the treatment of wounds; the plant herb was regularly used in America as a diuretic, sedative, and astringent, as well as to treat depression.

With the advent of the twentieth century, however,

conventional medicine and synthetic drugs held full sway in therapeutic arenas on both sides of the Atlantic Ocean. The practice of herbal medicine in English-speaking countries all but disappeared for more than fifty years, and with it was lost the popular use of St. John's wort. China and other Asian countries had, of course, held the practice of herbal medicine in high esteem for more than five thousand years, and the practice died harder there, only to regain renewed strength after the People's Revolution.

In the West, however, only non-English-speaking European countries, most notably Germany, still favored the therapeutic use of natural herbs over synthetic drugs whenever possible. In fact, in the late 1970s and throughout the 1980s it was Germany that gave us most of the seminal scientific research on the now well-established antidepressant properties of St. John's wort—and precipitated a scientific and media whirlwind in the process. British researchers soon confirmed the validity of Germany's successful and extensive use of St. John's wort for depression. American researchers followed with their own validating studies, and were quick to point out that they had been investigating the effectiveness of St. John's wort in treating AIDS, hepatitis, tuberculosis, cancer, and, most recently, obesity.

But it would be a mistake to think that conventional medicine's current serious interest in the use of St. John's wort has just now appeared, in the late 1990s. In fact, when the turbulent sixties ushered in a generation that demanded "alternative" choices for a variety of beliefs, practices, and systems, alternative medicine began its strong and steady comeback, and along with it came a renewed interest in herbal medicine—on both the younger generation's and the establishment's part.

Serious scientific investigation into the therapeutic properties of St. John's wort has been going on since at least the mid-1960s, when much of the focus was on its antibacterial properties. Antiviral research in general has been documented since the 1970s, and investigations into the use of St. John's wort to treat AIDS and several cancers began in the mid-1980s. Obesity studies are more recent, with one major clinical trial just completed in 1997 and another proposed for 1998.

That's an extraordinary road for one humble herb to have traveled, from the days when it was tossed into medieval bonfires to frighten away demons, to its current position as a possible breakthrough antiviral drug.

To appreciate how St. John's wort can have such a wide range of therapeutic properties and possibilities, we need to look a bit at the biology and chemistry of the plant itself. Chapter 2 describes the plant's botanical properties and chemical constituents.

CHAPTER 2

❖

The Magic of the Medicine

It purges choleric humours, helps the sciatica and gout, and heals burns. . . . It is a sovereign remedy for either wound or sore.

—NICHOLAS CULPEPER,
BRITISH APOTHECARY AND HERBALIST 1616–1654

GETTING TO KNOW THE PLANT

The Latin botanical name for St. John's wort, *Hypericum Perforatum* (or *H. Perforatum*), is commonly referred to in the lay literature simply as "hypericum." A perennial plant, hypericum is found throughout Europe, Asia, Australia, and the United States, and in all but the coldest and most northerly parts of the world. It grows wild along roadsides and riverbanks, in woods and fields—on virtually any open land—and prefers hard, dry, calcified soil. Hypericum is also readily grown by sowing its seeds in open ground, and requires little to no care.

The plant grows from June through August, but its flowers usually bloom in late June. After the flower petals fall off or are harvested, the plant naturally reseeds itself, lying dormant for the winter and then growing new shoots in the spring. Hypericum is one of a large family of herbaceous, shrub-like plants called *Hypericaceae* that includes more than 350 species. Some of the better known species are *H. augustifolia*, *H. maculatum*, *H. barbatum*, and *H. hirsutum*, but *H. perforatum* is by far the most widely used and intensely studied of the hypericum species.

The plant grows from one to three feet high and is topped by clusters of twenty-five to a hundred flowers. The five-petaled flowers are bright yellow and edged with tiny black dots, and the leaves are oblong or elliptical in shape, ranging in color from dark to pale green. The leaves also are covered with small black dots that appear translucent when held up to the light. As mentioned earlier, these dots were originally thought to be holes or perforations, hence the name *perforatum*. The black dots on both flowers and leaves are in fact minute glands from which the plant's medicinal red oil is extracted.

The stems of the plant are unique to *Hypericum perforatum* and distinguish the plant from other hypericum species. They are pale green, hollow, oval or cylindrical in shape, and have opposing horizontal ribs (a latter characteristic found in none of the other species).

Hypericum has a distinctly aromatic and balsamic odor that smells somewhat sweet and is mildly resinous and bittersweet to the taste. Medicinal extracts of hypericum are available in either fresh or dried form. All the above-ground (aerial) parts of the plant are used medicinally, including the buds, flowers, leaves, and stems. They are best harvested either right before the plant blooms or when it is in flower. (See Chapter 4 for more detailed information on harvesting, collection, and therapeutic forms of the herb.)

---------------------------- ❖ ----------------------------

Michael's Story: St. John's Wort's Success As a Stress-Buster

Michael uses St. John's wort preventively as a "stress-buster." He has found it to be powerfully effective in relieving the anxiety around his new and extremely stressful job in Hollywood's film industry.

Two years ago Michael left a highly successful career on Wall Street, where he was a top financial analyst, to resettle in Los Angeles and pursue a longtime dream of making independent films. At thirty-nine this was a gutsy move, but Michael was well prepared. He had spent more than three years studying filmmaking and he had saved a considerable amount of money over the last decade, knowing he would have to start at the bottom of the ladder in his new career.

Michael bought a small house in a suburb of Los Angeles, and through the fortuitous connections of several former Wall Street clients he got a job as assistant to an award-winning top independent filmmaker. Michael saw his new job as both an opportunity to break into the film business and a chance to learn at the feet of a master. What he didn't know, however, was that he was the director's sixth assistant in eighteen months!

"I thought the pressures of Wall Street had prepared me for anything," Michael says. "But Wall Street was a cakewalk compared to what goes on in the film business. Constant hustling, constant double-dealing, constant pressure from financial backers. The creative part of making films, the part I dreamed about for so long, gets overshadowed by the big business and the big egos behind the scenes. And nobody has a bigger ego than the man I work for. Still, I think I could have dealt with all that, given some time. But this man also turned out to be downright abusive. And that was something I'd never dealt with before."

Michael's new boss is what is known as a "screamer." He yells on the phone, he yells out his office door, he yells at assistants, he yells at the copy machine. Nothing

is ever done fast enough or well enough for him, and he
has no qualms about letting everyone know he's unhappy. Most mornings he storms into the office, in-
variably late, and marches right past Michael's desk
without even a hello. An air of gloom and terror often
emanates from his office. After a month of this behavior, Michael had a perpetual knot in his stomach, an intermittent tremor in his hands, trouble sleeping at night,
and a nearly uncontrollable urge to deck his boss—who
clearly wasn't going to change his ways.

"I really didn't want to quit my job. I'm not a quitter.
And I had just made a lot of sacrifices and burned quite
a few bridges to start all over again in L.A. Plus, I loved
the work and what I was learning, and I got along just
fine with the rest of the staff. But this guy was driving
me crazy, and I was afraid I'd be forced to quit. A lot of
the people on staff were popping Valium and Xanax
throughout the day to cope, but I've always been a bit
of a health nut, and I didn't want to go that route."

Michael was complaining about all this to his sister
over the phone one Friday night. A massage therapist,
his sister had been involved in alternative medicine for
over a decade. She knew several people who had been
prescribed St. John's wort for anxiety and insomnia,
and they'd been happy with the results. She suggested
Michael try it himself.

"I bought a bottle of the liquid extract at my local
health food shop that Saturday, and I took it to work
with me the following Monday. Later that morning,
when my boss stormed past me into his office, snapping
out some order on the way, I took out my St. John's
wort and put a dropperful under my tongue—about fifteen drops. Within half an hour I felt calmer, more centered, and more focused. I was able to let some of my

boss's abusive behavior slide more easily off my back. Then I had another dropperful in the afternoon, since that's when things really get crazy at my office. Again I experienced that feeling of calm and focus, but it wasn't a 'drugged' feeling at all. If anything, I was able to think more clearly and work more efficiently.

"I took St. John's wort like this for almost two weeks, and I noticed that not only was I able to handle the stress in the office better, but I was also sleeping well again and had a lot more energy. It's been six months since I started taking St. John's wort, and I don't use it every day now. Maybe two or three times a week, twice a day. But I always have it with me on the job. And it still helps me tremendously to deal with stress and stay focused on my tasks. In fact, it's become kind of an inside joke at my company. On my boss's worst days, when I can hear him begin to rant and rave in his office, I just take out my little brown bottle and wave it in the direction of his door. Then the other assistants know it's time to run for cover."

❖

GETTING TO KNOW
THE PLANT'S CONSTITUENTS

While all parts of the hypericum plant contain important chemical compounds—traditionally called the plant's "constituents"—the flowers and leaves are believed to yield the highest concentrations of hypericum's major constituents. And it is the therapeutic action of those major constituents, working singly and in combination, that is responsible for the plant's wide-ranging healing activities.

Current conventional research into hypericum's therapeutic properties has focused almost exclusively on the plant's individual constituents rather than on the plant's action as a whole. A basic knowledge of what those constituents are and how they act in the body is certainly fundamental to beginning to understand how and why hypericum is effective for such a diverse group of medical conditions. But first a caveat . . .

Focusing on the therapeutic actions of *single* constituents of hypericum is a dicey proposition at best. Such a focus implies that a medicinal plant can be neatly divided up into its most important "parts" and the specific therapeutic action of each part studied in isolation. The presumptive theory is that one and only one constituent of a plant is responsible, for example, for a plant's antiviral properties. The pharmaceutical scientist's goal is to isolate that constituent, synthesize it, and market it to the public in its "purest" and most therapeutically effective form.

This modern, purist approach to medicinal plants has never been embraced by traditional herbal medicine and is proving true only part of the time for conventional science. Take the example of hypericum's role as an antidepressant. Most current researchers admit that it's not entirely clear just how hypericum treats depression so effectively. And while most conventional research has focused on just two constituents of hypericum as the primary antidepressant agents (hypericin and pseudohypericin), some researchers now believe that other hypericum constituents are also critically involved in the process. Traditional practitioners would have assumed this from the outset. The two camps simply have different therapeutic perspectives when it comes to "drugs" and healing.

TWO DIVERSE PERCEPTIONS: THE WHOLE VS. THE PARTS

While conventional medicine and alternative medicine share similar goals—healing disease and promoting good health—their approach to healing is often markedly different, as is their view and use of drugs and herbs.

In treating an illness, the therapeutic approach of conventional medicine and pharmacology (the study of drugs) is generally militant, aggressive, and narrowly focused. The most biochemically effective single drug is identified to fight a specific disease. In the most simplistic terms, conventional medicine and pharmacology view the unhealthy body as a battlefield, with disease the enemy and drugs the weapons of war. Conventional medical language reflects that attitude: diseases are attacked; viruses are destroyed; illnesses are beaten; patients are victimized, lost, or saved. Far too often the disease is treated first, the person second, and the debris of the battle left for someone else to sweep away.

Make no mistake, the results of that kind of approach have frequently been stunning. Some viruses and bacteria that used to decimate humankind are virtually nonexistent. Still, the single-drug/single-disease approach often jeopardizes the body's overall health in the process. Secondary illnesses and dangerous or debilitating side effects are frequently the norm of single-drug therapies.

In contrast, alternative medicine's approach to disease is holistic. A person's illness is viewed as just one manifestation of a larger health imbalance. The illness is treated, of course, but so is the underlying imbalance, overall health, and general well-being. Special attention is always paid to offsetting side effects and avoiding the creation of new health problems in the bargain. It takes more than one plant constituent to do all that.

Thus the therapeutic focus of alternative medical practitioners who use medicinal plant herbs is the unique healing synergy of *all* the constituents in a plant. Plant herbs, and combinations of herbs (called herbal formulas), are prescribed not only to treat a specific illness, but also to simultaneously strengthen other systems in the body and reduce troublesome side effects. Since herbs are prescribed for their *collective* therapeutic action, it is less important to the practitioner what *part* of the herb works and more important that all the parts work well *together*.

Indeed, the alternative practitioner would be wary about using only a single-action herb constituent and would rightfully worry about what he or she was "losing" in overall healing benefits by separating the parts from the whole. In conventional medicine, separating the parts from the whole is nothing less than the beginning of good science. Each side has a point, but those who wonder what is lost in pursuit of good science sometimes have the edge.

An example from fairly recent medical history about the discovery and use of another "miracle" drug from the plant kingdom aptly illustrates this point.

THE GIFT OF THE MEADOWSWEET PLANT

When aspirin was "discovered" in 1899, it was roundly received as a nearly miraculous pharmaceutical breakthrough. It is an extraordinary drug indeed. Easy and economical to make, simple to take. It relieves pain, reduces inflammation, lowers fever, and, as recently discovered, promotes cardiovascular health and helps prevent heart attacks by acting as an anticlotting agent in the blood. Aspirin was a life raft, especially for those living with chronic pain.

But aspirin also has side effects, mostly gastrointestinal, ranging from mild stomach upsets to chronic and painful gastritis, from ulcers to potentially dangerous internal bleeding. Even moderate use of aspirin is believed to cause some internal bleeding. The drug also can interfere with the normal blood-clotting mechanism, and surgical patients are routinely warned not to take aspirin for at least a week before any surgery.

For people living with chronic pain—those with arthritis, for example—the regular use of aspirin became problematic after a while, despite its superior pain-relieving and anti-inflammatory properties, because of the potential for chronic stomach problems and internal bleeding. Those problems, in fact, were the primary reason that the ibuprofens or NSAIDs (nonsteroidal anti-inflammatory drugs) were created. Yet aspirin, as it was naturally found in plant herbs, didn't pose the same problems that its commercial form did. Quite the contrary.

Aspirin, a salicylic acid compound, was originally discovered as a constituent of the meadowsweet plant *(Filipendula ulmaria)*. In fact, aspirin gets it names from the former genus name of that plant, *Spiraea* (a *Spiraea* meaning "from meadowsweet"). What conventional science overlooked, or chose to ignore, when it isolated aspirin from meadowsweet is that traditional herbalists had been successfully using the entire meadowsweet plant for hundreds of years to relieve pain and inflammation, particularly that of arthritis and rheumatism, *and* to treat indigestion, acid stomach, and other gastrointestinal complaints! In the case of this plant herb, the whole *was* therapeutically greater than the parts.

❖

The whole of *Hypericum perforatum* also may prove to be far greater than any of its parts. Natural derivatives of the plant that retain as many of its vital constituents as possible are proving to have extraordinarily wide-ranging therapeutic effects.

And, in focusing on hypericum's constituents, the gift that conventional science offers should not be under-estimated. Not only are hypericum's many therapeutic uses being validated, one part at a time, but our understanding of how hypericum works has been immeasurably increased.

A BASIC PRIMER:
HYPERICUM'S CONSTITUENTS

The study of plant chemistry is called pharmacognosy or phytochemistry. It is an infinitely rich and complex science, because any one plant may contain hundreds of biologically active and inactive chemicals. Hypericum is no different and contains more than twenty active chemical compounds.

This primer on hypericum's constituents, therefore, is meant only to provide the bare basics about the known biological activities of a small group of the plant's chemical compounds—the ones that have been the subject of the most scientific scrutiny. Many of the references listed in the back of this book contain more complete discussions of plant chemistry in general and hypericum in particular.

The classes of constituents and chemical compounds that have been studied most intensely are listed below, followed by a brief description highlighting their traditional medicinal uses and those primary therapeutic actions that have been substantiated by modern research.

HYPERICUM'S PRIMARY CONSTITUENTS

QUINONES
- hypericin
- pseudohypericin

FLAVONOIDS
- hyperin
- quercitin
- biflavone
- proanthocyanidin
- amentoflavone

ESSENTIAL/VOLATILE OILS

XANTHONES

TANNINS

COUMARINS
- Umbelliferone
- Scopoletin

QUINONES

The quinones are one of several classes of plant constituents that have the acidic phenol compounds as the fundamental building blocks of their chemical structure. Naturally occurring pigments, the quinones are red, yellow, or orange benzene-based chemical compounds. Some have biological importance as coenzymes and vitamins, others as hydrogen receptors. Traditionally, the quinones have antiseptic, antibacterial, anti-inflammatory, and analgesic actions.

The quinones **hypericin** and **pseudohypericin** are photosensitive, naturally occurring red pigments currently considered to be the most biologically significant extracts of the hypericum plant. Both constituents have been the primary focus of most clinical research in recent years, with hypericin—in its natural or synthetic form—being the most frequently studied of the two.

Hypericin and pseudohypericin are found throughout the hypericum plant, but are most highly concentrated in the flower petals and buds. Since both constituents, and especially hypericin extracts, have generated a substantial body of research, we are summarizing their therapeutic actions by those properties that have been the most intensely studied.

Antiviral Properties. *In vitro* studies (in test tube or other artificial environment) have confirmed that both hypericin and pseudohypericin have powerful antiviral properties against the herpes simplex viruses I and II, Epstein-Barr virus, influenzas A and B, vesicular stomatitis virus, and equine infectious anemia virus. Most significantly, hypericin and pseudohypericin have demonstrated potent antiviral activity against the HIV virus responsible for AIDS, with studies having been conducted both *in vitro* and in animals and humans *(in vivo)*. The antiviral activity of both hypericin and pseudohypericin is substantially enhanced in the presence of light (photoactivation).

Anticancer Properties. Hypericin has been tested *in vitro* as an anticancer agent against breast cancer and several skin cancers, and in patients with glioma, the most common and most deadly form of brain cancer. Hypericin demonstrated significant anticancer properties in two ways: at low doses it inhibited the growth of new cancer cells; at high doses it killed cancer cells. Compared with Tamoxifen, a standard chemotherapeutic drug used to treat both breast cancer and glioma, hypericin's effectiveness was equal to or even greater than Tamoxifen's, and it was less toxic and better tolerated. Hypericin also has demonstrated effectiveness against the skin cancer melanoma, both alone and as an adjunctive therapy with laser treatment.

Antidepressant Properties. Clinical studies of the effectiveness of hypericin and pseudohypericin, in natural or synthetic forms, have dominated contemporary research for the last fifteen years and garnered the most scientific and popular attention. However, it is still unclear just how and why hypericin and pseudohypericin—along with other constituents of hypericum—work as antidepressants. It appears that they act both as mild monoamine oxidase inhibitors (MAOIs) and strong serotonin reuptake inhibitors (SRIs).

What is clear, from both *in vitro* studies of hypericin and pseudohypericin and clinical trials involving more than 5,000 patients, is that they are significantly effective in treating the symptoms of mild to moderately severe depression, including sadness, decreased energy, fatigue, insomnia, and irritability. Both hypericin and pseudohypericin have far fewer side effects than standard antidepressants, and they are considerably less expensive to make and to buy.

Some research has suggested that the antidepressant action of these two constituents is enhanced by the fact that they also are immune-stimulators and thus relieve many of the physical symptoms associated with depression while strengthening the body's defense system overall. Still other researchers have proposed the theory that hypericin and pseudohypericin may not be the only constituents responsible for hypericum's antidepressant effectiveness. In fact, some of hypericum's flavonoids, as well as its xanthones, have exhibited stronger MAO-inhibiting properties.

FLAVONOIDS

The flavonoids, among the most common of plant constituents, are phenol compounds found in the highest concentrations in plants with yellow-colored fruits, flowers, and leaves. They have a wide range of traditional therapeutic indications and have been variously used as diuretics, antispasmodics, anti-inflammatories, antibacterials, antivirals, and antifungals. There is some evidence that they also have anticancer properties. The flavonoids are particularly useful for problems of the circulatory system and are known to both lower blood pressure and strengthen blood capillaries. In hypericum, the highest concentrations of flavonoids are found in the flowers of the plant.

Five hypericum flavonoids have demonstrated impressive and varied therapeutic actions in conventional research studies: **hyperin** and **biflavone** as sedatives; **quericitin** as an MAO inhibitor; **proanthocyanidin** as a vasorelaxant, antioxidant, antiviral, and antibacterial; and **amentoflavone** as an anti-inflammatory, sedative, and inhibitor of ulcer development.

ESSENTIAL OILS

The essential oils are what give a plant its distinctive smell, and thus they are widely used commercially in perfumes and other scented products. Other than that, the essential oils have been generally underinvestigated by conventional science.

In traditional herbal medicine, however, the essential oils of plants have wide-ranging therapeutic uses. They have been prescribed variously as antiseptics, antispasmodics, antifungals, antidepressants, digestive aids, mood elevators, pain relievers, and sedatives. In Chinese herbal medicine, many plant oils are especially esteemed for their ability to induce sweat and reduce fevers.

There are five basic chemical groups of essential oils—the monoterpenes, sesquiterpenes, diterpenes, sesterterpenes, and triterpenes. Hypericum's essential oils primarily contain monoterpenes and sesquiterpenes, with the highest concentrations found in all but the stem of the plant at the time the plant is just beginning to flower.

The monoterpenes are noted for their antifungal properties and for stimulating the circulatory system. Many also have sedating and calming effects on the central nervous system.

The sesquiterpenes are antiseptic, anti-inflammatory, and antispasmodic, and may be effective in treating simple anxiety, tension, and headaches. They also are indicated for the treatment of hay fever and allergic asthma.

Recent research into the therapeutic properties of hypericum's essential oils have confirmed their sedating and antifungal properties.

XANTHONES

The xanthones are aromatic, naturally occurring yellow pigments that constitute a subgroup of the flavonoids called flavonoid aglycones. Like their parent group, they have anti-inflammatory, antispasmodic, antiseptic, and diuretic actions. They also are considered excellent tonics for the circulatory system. In the hypericum plant, the highest concentration of xanthones is found in the flowers.

Over the last ten years research into the therapeutic properties of hypericum's xanthones has confirmed their diuretic and cardiotonic properties, and further demonstrated that they are antidepressant, antibacterial, antiviral, and MAO-inhibiting.

TANNINS

The tannins are another subgroup of the large phenol class, best known for their use in tanning (browning and hardening) animal skins. Therapeutically, they have a much wider range of use. Basically astringent in nature, the tannins have been used externally to heal wounds and burns and to reduce inflammations. Internally, they are used to stop diarrhea and internal bleeding.

Research has confirmed that the tannins in hypericum are antidiarrheal. The tannins, found in highest concentrations in the leaves and flowers during the plant's blossoming period, are no doubt significant agents in the plant's historically well-known effectiveness as a wound healer, as they dry and bind skin.

COUMARINS

The coumarins, also a subgroup of the large phenol class, are benzopyrone derivatives. They are found throughout the hypericum plant, but mostly in the leaves and flowers. In other plants, the coumarins are strongly aromatic; in fact, they are the chemicals responsible for the rich scent of new-mown hay given off by cut grass. Traditionally, coumarins have been used for their antibacterial and antifungal actions.

Conventional medicine has long used a coumarin derivative called dicumarol as the basis for the powerful anti-blood clotting agent, warfarin—though coumarins are traditionally not used for this indication in herbal medicine. (In large doses, dicumarol/warfarin are toxic and, in fact, used as rat poison.)

Current research has identified the therapeutic actions of two other coumarin derivatives: **umbelliferone** and **scopoletin**, which have anti-inflammatory, antifungal, and *in vitro* antitumor properties.

Other Hypericum Constituents and Their Therapeutic Properties

Several other constituents of hypericum have documented therapeutic effects. **Hyperforin** and **adhyperforin**, two phloroglucinols, have demonstrated significant antibacterial and wound-healing properties. In one study, both constituents were stronger than standard sulfur drugs. Hyperforin is highly effective against the notorious "staph" infection, *Staphyloccus aureus bacteria,* which routinely plagues hospitals and clinics. There is evidence that it also may have anticancer properties.

Hypericum also contains **carotenoids**, which are believed to enhance the plant's burn-healing mechanism by increasing the amount of oxygen available in the body.

Several amino acids are found in hypericum, most notably **gamma-aminobutyric acid** (GABA), a transmitter of nerve impulses in the central nervous system that some research indicates has sedating effects.

Hypericum also contains **beta-sitosterol**, a known estrogenic compound, though this constituent seems to have received little attention. It may, however, have some therapeutic role in hypericum's traditional use as a treatment for menstrual and menopausal symptoms.

THE WHOLE PLANT: A SUPER ANTIBACTERIAL AND ANTIBIOTIC

As mentioned in the first chapter, extracts from the hypericum plant's flower and leaves traditionally have been used for a variety of therapeutic actions—anti-inflammatory, astringent, analgesic, antispasmodic, diuretic, sedating, and vulnerary. It is as a superior vulnerary—a wound healer—that hypericum has been most celebrated through the centuries.

Research studies over the last thirty years have confirmed hypericum's antibacterial and antibiotic properties. Externally, it effectively treats wounds, burns, and several other skin conditions. Internally, it has proven effectiveness *in vitro* and *in vivo* against tuberculosis, staph, colitis, candida, shigella, and infections of the urinary tract, ear, and throat.

Hypericum appears to fight bacterial infections in two ways. First, its strong antiseptic and antibacterial properties kill germs outright. Second, research indicates that several hypericum constituents work directly on the immune system, both decreasing inflammations related to the immune-response and increasing the body's ability to fight off the infection.

❖

MOVING FORWARD

This has been a very general overview of the therapeutic properties of St. John's wort. Still, it is quite clear that this much-esteemed plant has tremendous applications for healing—many of which are just now being tapped by conventional medicine, but all of which have long been practiced by alternative healers.

Indeed, St. John's wort seems to be an effective and practical alternative to many synthetic pharmaceuticals, and it is widely available, safe to use, and far less expensive than prescription drugs. We discuss just how safe St. John's wort is in the next chapter, and then describe how to find and buy the herb itself. Part II of the book describes the many practical healing applications for St. John's wort, based on its known therapeutic actions.

For now, let's end with a bow to the apothecary, Nicholas Culpeper, with whom we began this chapter. Angry and tired with the monopoly on medical care that Britain's College of Physicians exerted, Culpeper took it upon himself in 1649 to translate the college's *Pharma-*

copoeia from Latin to English. The new translation became the famous Culpeper *Herbal*, and it made the *Pharmacopoeia*'s vast store of knowledge about healing herbs available to the very people who couldn't afford doctors to begin with, England's working poor.

In many ways, the maverick and much-maligned Culpeper was the key to galvanizing the public's and conventional medicine's attention on the power of Western herbal medicine, and the fact that it was a medicine for the people first and foremost. And he did it 350 years ago.

CHAPTER 3

❖

Is St. John's Wort for Everyone?

One hundred and five outpatients with mild depression of short duration were treated with either hypericum extract or placebo. The therapy phase was four weeks. In the hypericum group, 67% of patients responded to treatment compared to 28% in the placebo group. Notable side effects were not found.
—JOURNAL OF GERIATRIC PSYCHIATRY AND NEUROLOGY
(OCTOBER 1994, SUPPLEMENT)

In this chapter we look at two critical yet under-discussed areas surrounding hypericum: the side effects associated with its use, and those situations where it shouldn't be used at all. The popular press and some recent books seem to suggest that hypericum is so benign that it is suitable for just about anyone and any situation. This simply isn't true.

Let's start our discussion, then, by addressing the question "Is St. John's wort for everyone?" The answer is an unequivocal "no." Plant herbs are medicine, and any medication—whether prescription or over the counter, natural or synthetic—carries with it some inherent risks. Hypericum is no different.

Many people mistakenly assume that because plant herbs are natural they are automatically safe, or certainly safer than many synthetic prescription drugs. This can be a dangerous, even fatal, assumption. In some cases, in fact, the reverse is true. For example, a chemical constituent of the foxglove plant *(Digitalis purpurea)* provided the medical world with one of its most powerful drugs for treating heart failure—digitalis. But the foxglove plant itself is poisonous. The deadly nightshade plant *(Atropa belladonna)*—

"deadly" is part of its actual name, by the way—offered up atropine, the basic chemical constituent of many drugs, belladonna among them, that soothe painful muscle spasms. This plant, too, is poisonous. The beautiful white poppy *(Papaver somniferum)* gave us morphine, an invaluable drug for relieving excruciating and debilitating pain, especially the pain experienced by many of the terminally ill. It also gave us heroin, one of our most deadly drugs of abuse. Because of their possible threat, none of these herbs is listed in popular books on Western herbalism, despite the value of some of their chemical components.

Hypericum is not even remotely related to the poisonous plants. And yet its general safety was the subject of some controversy as recently as 1984, when it was listed in *American Pharmacy* as one of several "dangerous herbs," partly due to effects observed in animals who grazed on it in large quantities. This information proved to be erroneous when hypericum was used by people in normal doses, but it underscores an important point we want to make in this chapter: Approach all medicine, whatever its origin, with respect and healthy skepticism.

Developing a healthy skepticism is especially important with regard to hypericum since a wealth of new research studies are currently under way that focus on the herb's therapeutic applications for a wide variety of disorders. The information released from these studies, usually in encapsulated form, can be both exciting and confusing. Learning how to critically read the results of those studies and apply them to your personal situation is crucial to making an informed decision about using hypericum.

This is particularly important if you are thinking of using hypericum for depression, currently its most popular application. We discuss depression in more detail in Chapter 5, but it is worth repeating here the proviso that depression is a serious medical illness. Any depression must be thoroughly assessed, diagnosed, and treated. Any treatment for it must be carefully monitored. Some depressions don't respond to some antidepressants, hypericum among them. No doubt hypericum is a very effective antidepressant for many types of depressions—and an equally effective treatment for several other disorders. But many popular reports on St. John's wort, including the "abridged" versions of medical studies often included in those reports, make hypericum sound like a magical panacea for myriad illnesses, depression among them. In the end, hypericum is medicine, not magic. And as more information on this astounding plant herb is published, you need to know not only about side effects and contraindications, but also how to separate the fact from fantasy.

So before we move on to hypericum's side effects and contraindications, let's briefly look at how to be a healthy skeptic.

How to Be a Healthy Skeptic

We chose the paraphrased excerpt that starts this chapter for two reasons.

First, the *Journal of Geriatric Psychiatry and Neurology* is a highly respected medical journal. The October 1994 supplemental issue where this abstract appeared did much to focus serious medical and public attention on St. John's wort. The entire issue is devoted to articles featuring clinical studies of hypericum and its effectiveness in treating depression and several other disorders. This issue contains much excellent information on hypericum's therapeutic properties and on side effects encountered during the various treatment studies.

Second, the excerpt we quote has also been cited in

other books and articles about hypericum as substantiation of the herb's effectiveness and safety. In particular, the fact that no "notable side effects" were found is often cited. Let's look at that excerpt again: "One hundred and five outpatients with mild depression of short duration were treated with either hypericum extract or placebo. The therapy phase was four weeks. In the hypericum group, 67% of patients responded to treatment compared to 28% in the placebo group. Notable side effects were not found."

Here are some of the questions we would ask after reading this abstract—and that you should ask as a healthy skeptic—in an attempt to understand how safe and effective hypericum really is for personal use:

❖ *Who were these patients? What were their ages and genders? What other illnesses did they have, if any? Were they taking any other medications? How was improvement in depression measured?*

The patients ranged in age from 20 to 65 years old and were mostly female. They were otherwise healthy, and though some were on other medications, the researchers reported no drug interactions with hypericum. Of note is the fact that the results reported in this study were for 89 people only—not 105, as the text of the journal article implies. Seven people were excluded before the study began because their symptoms had changed. Nine other people dropped out of the study for various reasons. By the study's end, there were 42 patients in the hypericum group, 28 (67%) of whom showed significant improvement, and there were 47 patients in the placebo group, only 13 (28%) of whom showed an improvement. Improvement was measured by comparing patient scores on the Hamilton Depression Rating Scale (a standard psychiatric assessment tool), which was administered at the start of the study, two weeks into the study, and at the end of the study.

❖ **What is a mild depression? What is a mild depression of short duration? Do those labels apply to me and my situation?**

These patients had been diagnosed with mild "neurotic" depression that didn't interfere significantly with family and work life. Their symptoms had only been present for a brief time and included depressed mood, disturbed sleep, anxiety, headache, and fatigue, among others. The researchers themselves recommended that hypericum not be used for more serious depressions that involve suicidal thoughts and/or interfere with family and work.

❖ **How much hypericum was used and how often? What's a placebo?**

This was in fact an Austrian study—though it was reported in an American medical journal—and the hypericum extract used was a European formulation called Jarsin 300. Patients took three doses of 300 mg each daily for a total of 900 mg of hypericum daily, a standard hypericum treatment regimen for mild-to-moderate depression.

However, most clinical studies report using hypericum extract that is standardized to 0.3% hypericin. Therefore, three 300 mg doses per day of hypericum extract contain a total of 0.9% or almost 1 mg of hypericin. As we mentioned in Chapter 1, hypericin is the primary chemical constituent of hypericum and the one believed to contain much of the herb's antidepressive properties. To ensure the herb's quality and therapeutic potency, all hypericum extract should contain at least 0.3% hypericin, and most commercially available hypericum is indeed standardized to 0.3% hypericin. (See Chapter 4 for more information about various hypericum formulations.)

However, the hypericum extract used in this study, Jarsin 300, was standardized to 0.9% hypericin for a total daily dose of 2.7 mg of hypericin, considerably higher than most medical practitioners recommend for long-term treatment of mild to moderate depression. What is of special interest here is that even at more potent levels, hypericum still produced very mild side effects. In fact, strangely enough, hypericum users had far fewer and milder side effects than did the placebo users.

A placebo is a "dummy" pill used in clinical trials that study the effectiveness of a new "drug." The placebo pill looks identical to the real drug being studied, but there is no medication in a placebo (often it just contains sugar). By comparing a new drug's effectiveness against a placebo drug, researchers can be reasonably assured that any effects they observe in patients during a study are indeed due to the new drug's therapeutic properties. The fact that some patients (13 in this study) showed some kind of improvement on a "dummy" drug is known as the "placebo effect." That is, some patients' symptoms improve just by virtue of their *thinking* they're getting medication for them.

The irony in this study is that the placebo patients had far more side effects (see "side effects," below) than did the patients who actually received medication. This may be partly because the placebo patients were receiving no treatment for their depressive symptoms.

❖ *Why did therapy last only four weeks? Should I be on hypericum for only four weeks?*

Four and six weeks are standard but "artificial" treatment times used in clinical studies that focus on measuring the initial therapeutic effects of a new drug compared to another drug or placebo. The real treatment of depression, however, is longer term. Usually a minimum of a year of using the medication is required. Taking hypericum for depression for only four weeks would be ineffective. In fact, most studies indicate that it takes at least ten days to two weeks for hypericum to begin to take effect at all.

❖ *What's a "notable side effect"? If notable side effects weren't found, were other less notable side effects found? If so, what were they and how many people experienced them?*

Notable side effects would include those that were so severe or uncomfortable that they necessitated either medical attention or a patient to stop taking the study drug. No such effects were reported in this study. In fact, only two patients taking hypericum reported bothersome side effects: one patient had reddening of the skin and another experienced fatigue. Three patients in the placebo group reported side effects that included stomach pain, sleepiness, weight gain, and fluid retention.

What Can We Assume from This Study?

All we can reasonably assume from this single study is that for a small group of people (28 out of 42 patients taking hypericum at standard daily doses), there was a significant improvement in some symptoms of mild depression, ranging from relief of depressed moods and anxiety to better sleep patterns and increased energy. Furthermore, side effects were few and relatively mild. For this small group of people, hypericum was certainly safe *and* effective.

But can we also make the assumption that therefore

hypericum is safe for most people? Not from this small study alone. Fortunately for us, several large-scale studies have monitored hypericum's safety in more than 5,000 patients, and the good results obtained are similar to those found in the smaller study.

So Is Hypericum Safe?

For most people and for most situations, in doses of up to 900 mg a day, substantial clinical evidence suggests that hypericum is generally safe and causes few side effects. Those side effects that do occur are relatively mild and short-lasting.

The largest drug-monitoring study of hypericum's safety and effectiveness was conducted in 1993 among 3,250 German patients who received hypericum extract for four weeks. The hypericum formulation used in this trial was the same as in the smaller study we have just discussed (Jarsin 300, also called LI 160). Patients took 300 mg of hypericum, standardized to 0.9% hypericin, three times a day, for a daily total of 900 mg hypericum containing 2.7 mg of hypericin.

The patients ranged in age from 20 to 90, with an average age of 51 years, and 76% of patients were females. Almost half of the patients (49%) had mild depression, and another 46% had intermediate or moderate depression. A small group of patients (3%) were severely depressed.

Only 79 patients (2.4%) in the entire study experienced side effects. Among this group of patients, the major side effects reported were gastrointestinal upsets (18 patients), including nausea, stomach pain, and diarrhea; allergic reactions (17 patients), including skin rashes; fatigue (13 patients); anxiety or restlessness (8 patients); and dizziness (5 patients).

Similar side effects were reported in a second drug-monitoring study. In 1996, the *British Medical Journal* published a retrospective meta-analysis of twenty-three smaller studies that used hypericum extract to treat depression. A combined total of 1,757 patients with mild-to-moderate depression received various hypericum extracts (no one formulation was used); the effectiveness and safety of hypericum were then compared to either a placebo or a standard antidepressant. In this meta-analysis, the rate of side effects for hypericum was higher than in the larger study described above. Fifty patients (19.8%) reported experiencing side effects similar to those found in the larger study. Still, this was significantly superior to the side effect rate found among patients taking standard antidepressants, 84 of whom (52.8%) reported experiencing adverse and more severe reactions to their medications.

—————————— ❖ ——————————

Sarah's Story: Mending Depression, Ending Cravings

The most recently discovered—and perhaps most intriguing—therapeutic benefit of St. John's wort is its apparent ability to help fight obesity and control weight. As discussed in Chapter 9, at least two clinical studies have just been conducted specifically to investigate the use of St. John's wort as a weight-loss aid, but most people first discovered this benefit of the herb while taking it for depression. Sarah, a twenty-eight-year-old research assistant, was one of them.

"I've been taking St. John's wort for mild depression for about five months now, nine hundred milligrams a day. The results have been astonishing. Not only do I deal with stressful situations far better, but I think more clearly and my creativity quotient seems to have doubled! I also sleep better and have a lot more energy. But the most surprising effect was that my appetite changed dramatically after about six weeks. For one thing, I didn't crave coffee anymore and, in fact, I gave up caffeine entirely. And it was easy. I also stopped craving fatty foods and sweets, and for the first time began to crave fruits and vegetables! Needless to say, when I started to eat more healthful foods, I began to lose weight. I don't know if this is a direct result of taking St. John's wort, but that's the only real change I made in my life in the last six months?!"

❖

The results from these two large drug-monitoring studies, together with information gathered in numerous smaller studies, generally indicate that four common side effects may be associated with the use of hypericum. In order of frequency and intensity, they are (1) gastrointestinal upsets; (2) allergic reactions, skin rashes, and photosensitivity; (3) fatigue; and (4) anxiety and/or restlessness.

Before we move on to take a brief look at each of these side effects and what you might do to alleviate them, a caution is in order. On an individual-by-individual basis, it may be difficult to identify these "side effects" as reactions to hypericum alone. They are also frequently among the "symptoms" of many of the medical conditions hypericum is used to treat, including depression, insomnia, anxiety, PMS, and menstrual and menopausal problems.

Remember, too, that these side effects have been reported by only a small number of people. In the large drug-monitoring study of more than 3,000 patients, only 18 reported having any gastrointestinal problems. Further, many of the side effects reported appear to be associated with the start of hypericum therapy. Side effects may disappear with continued use. Of course, if serious side effects occur, you should stop taking hypericum immediately. And again, we strongly advise you to work with a qualified medical practitioner if you decide to use hypericum for any medical problem. In the end, you are the best judge of how your body is feeling and how it reacts to treatment, but a practitioner can help you make adjustments in formulations and dosages, if necessary, and may suggest other alternative therapies to support your self-care regimen.

HYPERICUM'S SIDE EFFECTS AND HOW TO DEAL WITH THEM

- **Gastrointestinal Upsets.** A number of people taking hypericum report feeling nauseous or experiencing stomach pain, diarrhea, and appetite loss. Taking hypericum with, or just after, meals often alleviates this problem. You may also have to experiment with different formulations. (See Chapter 4 and the "Resources" section in the back of the book.) For example, some people tolerate the capsules better than they do the liquid extract—and vice versa. Some liquid extracts contain alcohol, which itself is upsetting to the stomach, but there are nonalcoholic formulations available as alternatives. And always dilute the liquid extract in a glass of spring water.

    Instead of taking hypericum three times a day with meals, which is most frequently recommended, you might try taking it in smaller doses throughout the day with meals and snacks, as long as your doses add up to the recommended total daily intake of no more than 900 mgs. This is easy to do if you are taking the liquid extract. Just decrease the number of drops you take at one time (usually 20 drops in water, three times a day) to 12 drops, five times a day. For capsule forms, look for the 300 mg scored tablets (see "Resources") which can easily be broken in half, and take 6 half-tablets evenly spaced throughout the day with meals and snacks.

This is also an optimal time to pay attention to good nutrition and proper sleep habits. Try eliminating foods and beverages that may irritate the stomach, and make rest and relaxation top priorities in your daily self-care regimen.

- **Allergic Reactions, Skin Rashes, and Photosensitivity.** Anyone can have an allergic reaction to just about any substance, hypericum included. Although no serious allergic reaction has ever been reported among hypericum users, there is always the small possibility that this may happen. If you should develop signs of a severe allergic reaction—hives, difficult breathing, facial swelling—seek medical attention immediately.

The "allergic reactions" reported in the large drug-monitoring study discussed above (largely skin rashes, irritation, and skin reddening) were experienced by only 13 patients. A number of these may have been bonafide mild allergic reactions to hypericum. However, they also may have been the result of one of hypericum's most publicized and least understood properties: the fact that it can act as a photosensitizing agent.

Hypericin, the primary chemical constituent of hypericum, is a significant photosensitizer. When taken in large quantities it can cause extreme sensitivity to sunlight and a condition called erythema, abnormal redness of the skin. This is rarely a problem in humans taking normal doses of hypericum, though it frequently has been reported as occurring in animals who graze on St. John's wort in large quantities.

Some very fair individuals may be more susceptible to sunburn while taking hypericum, and they are routinely advised to wear sunscreen and other skin and head protection, particularly in warmer or tropical climates. Fair-complexioned men who regularly work out-of-doors may also be more susceptible to sunburns and skin irritations while on hypericum and should take appropriate precautions. Additionally, some patients in clinical trials that used higher daily doses of hypericum (1,800 mg a day or more) and/or pure synthetic hypericin experienced both erythema and facial pain when they were exposed to sunlight. These effects were characterized as mild and transient, and they disappeared completely as soon as the hypericum was stopped.

Again, when hypericum is taken internally at recommended doses of up to 900 mg total a day, standardized to 0.3% hypericin, this is rarely a problem. It is worth mentioning, however, that hypericum's photosensitizing effect may be stronger when it is used topically (externally) on the skin and the patient is subsequently exposed to direct sunlight for any length of time.

In one rare case, a patient with a sprained ankle was treated with a combination of hypericum gel and ultrasound therapy. After treatment, the patient was working outdoors and developed second-degree burns that resulted in significant scarring. Another patient, treated in a similar manner with topical hypericum, also experienced extensive burning. These are very rare cases, but we mention them because several skin-care creams currently on the market have St. John's wort in them. We have at least one anecdotal report from a woman who received a free sample of such a cream, used it without knowing it contained St. John's wort, and experienced severe reddening of the skin when she went outdoors.

Since hypericum's photosensitizing effect is largely dose-related and may be particularly pronounced when the herb is used topically, you would do well to check the hypericum and hypericin contents of any hypericum oils or creams you intend to use.

- **Fatigue.** Thirteen patients in the large drug-monitoring study reported feeling significant fatigue, a side effect that also has been documented in several smaller studies. This is another reported "side effect" of hypericum that is difficult to distinguish from a bonafide symptom of the disorder being treated. The vast majority of information available about hypericum's side effects has been gathered almost exclusively in studies of its effectiveness in treating depression. This is a debilitating illness, physically and emotionally, with sleep disturbances and associate fatigue common symptoms.

  However, we now also know that several of hypericum's chemical constituents have mild sedating properties, and in fact the herb has traditionally been used—and recently been tested—as an aid for insomnia.

  The fatigue associated with hypericum use seems to be very transitory. In fact, most people report feeling *energized* after several weeks of taking the herb. For the small number of people who do experience troubling fatigue when first starting on hypericum, eliminating caffeine and nicotine, as well as adding some moderate exercise to one's daily self-care regimen, can go a long way toward achieving a good night's rest.

- **Anxiety and/or Restlessness.** Only 8 people out of more than 3,000 included in the large drug-monitoring study (discussed above) reported feeling anxious and/or restless while taking hypericum. Minimal as it is, this effect also has been reported in smaller studies.

    Initial anxiety and/or restlessness is a commonly reported side effect of most antidepressant treatment, particularly of the selective serotonin reuptake inhibitors (SSRIs) such as Prozac. As mentioned in Chapter 2, hypericum's antidepressant actions most resemble those of the SSRIs, though it has several other antidepressant properties as well, which we discuss in greater detail in Chapter 5. It is not clear why anxiety would be a side effect of a clearly anti-anxiety medication, such as hypericum. The good news is that these particular effects are quite transitory and usually disappear within the first two weeks of starting hypericum treatment. The better news is that more than 90% of all people who take hypericum never experience initial anxiety or restlessness.

❖

HYPERICUM'S CONTRAINDICATIONS: WHEN NOT TO USE HYPERICUM AND WHEN TO PROCEED WITH CAUTION

There now is a substantial body of serious clinical work documenting hypericum's excellent safety record, both in terms of side effects and interactions with other drugs, and in use with preexisting medical conditions. Generally, this research shows that under the supervision of a medical practitioner, hypericum is very safe in standard doses: it doesn't interact with other medications, with the possible exception of standard antidepressants (see Chapter 5 for more details), and it shouldn't pose a problem in people with chronic medical conditions, such as heart, kidney, and liver disease.

These clinical data are also supported by the extensive anecdotal and "real-life" information available from thousands of German physicians who have prescribed hypericum for millions of people for more than a decade. Among German patients, hypericum has a long and successful track record as a very safe drug.

Still, many people—and most conventional medical practitioners—want hard-core scientific evidence of a drug's efficacy and safety. So it's important to point out here—especially in a book that looks at hypericum's wide-ranging treatment applications—that most of the human safety information gathered about hypericum is from studies of *depressed* patients only. Further, those patients either were carefully monitored throughout hypericum treatment or were included in the studies because they *didn't* have other medical conditions or *weren't* taking other prescription drugs.

On paper and in controlled clinical trials, hypericum looks very safe. In actuality, it probably is very safe. In the popular press, several authors even suggest that hypericum is safe for pregnant women and young children (neither of whom it's ever been tested on!). But most medical practitioners, conventional and alternative, prefer to take a more cautious approach with hypericum, and there is a standard set of guidelines for when it should be used with caution and when it shouldn't be used at all. This is another reason why throughout this book we repeatedly recommend that you take hypericum—for whatever condition—only in partnership with a qualified medical practitioner.

Let's first look at those situations where hypericum shouldn't be used.

When Not to Use Hypericum

- Do not use hypericum if you are taking any kind of prescription antidepressant, particularly one of the selective serotonin reuptake inhibitors, such as Prozac. A potentially serious drug interaction called *serotonin syndrome* may occur if you do. We discuss depression and using hypericum for depression in greater detail in Chapter 5. We also offer suggestions about how to switch from a prescription antidepressant to hypericum, but this should only be done under the care of a qualified medical practitioner. If you are taking a prescription antidepressant and also want to try hypericum for another medical condition—PMS or insomnia, for example— please talk with a practitioner first. Do not self-medicate with hypericum if you are already taking a prescription antidepressant.

- Do not take hypericum for bipolar disorder (manic-depression) or severe depression that involves suicidal thoughts. Although some recent research suggests that higher daily doses of hypericum (1,800 mg or more per day) may be effective in treating more severe depressions, significantly more research is needed to justify those claims. Right now, hypericum is only indicated for mild to moderate depression and for seasonal affective disorder (SAD).

- Do not take hypericum if you are pregnant or nursing, despite the anecdotal information you may read in some popular literature about its longtime safe use by thousands of German women. Hypericum has never been tested for possible teratogenicity, that is, drug-caused genetic malformations in fetuses. Further, hypericum has a long traditional use as a uterine tonic and mild uterine stimulant; at least one contemporary study has verified its mild uterine-stimulating property in laboratory animals. (See Chapter 6 for a detailed discussion of St. John's wort as a "female" tonic.)

- Do not treat children under the age of 12 with topically (externally) applied hypericum, despite what you might read in some older herbals. For example, there is a long-standing and apparently effective traditional use of hypericum as a treatment for colicky babies. The baby is submerged in warm bathwater to which fresh hypericum (flowers and leaves) or liquid extract has been added. As mentioned in Chapter 2, hypericum has antispasmodic, analgesic, and sedating properties—all of which are useful in treating colic. A hypericum bath also is an excellent treatment for anxiety, restlessness, and stomach cramping. (In fact, we recommend it in Chapter 5 for women experiencing PMS and menstrual or menopausal problems.) But we don't recommend hypericum in any form for very young children. No research trials have studied hypericum's safety or effectiveness in youngsters, and they are especially sensitive to both the therapeutic and adverse effects of medications, be they natural or synthetic. Given the severe, albeit rare, skin reactions we described above when hypericum was used topically in a small group of adults, its use should definitely be avoided in young children.

- Do not use hypericum if you have a substance-abuse problem (with alcohol, cocaine, crack, heroin, or amphetamines). A serious drug interaction may occur, despite some anecdotal reports that hypericum is an effective "de-tox" medication. Instead, work with a qualified practitioner, counselor, or 12-Step group to get and stay sober. Then consider taking hypericum during the recovery phase, to treat related anxiety and insomnia.

When to Use Hypericum with Caution

- Use hypericum with caution and only under a qualified medical practitioner's care if you have chronic heart, liver, or kidney disease, or if you have been diagnosed with a connective tissue disease, such as lupus or rheumatoid arthritis. In chronic organ diseases, the body's defense mechanisms are severely compromised and often cannot effectively metabolize many medicines, botanical medicines included. People with heart, liver, and kidney disease are especially susceptible to serious drug-related side effects, even with a mild medicine such as hypericum. In connective tissue diseases, such as systemic lupus, photosensitivity and severe sun-related skin reactions are actual symptoms of the disease. Self-medicating with hypericum, a known photosensitizing plant herb, might seriously exacerbate these symptoms.

- Use hypericum with caution, and only under a practitioner's care, if you have chronic high blood pressure. (Also see the "Cautionary Endnote" below.)

- Use hypericum with caution, and only under a practitioner's care, if you have AIDS, cancer, or hepatitis, or have been diagnosed with HIV or tuberculosis. There has been much exciting news about hypericum's anti-viral, anticancer, antibacterial, and immune-boosting properties. Several studies are currently under way— and many more planned—to test hypericum's effectiveness in treating patients with AIDS, HIV, several of the hepatitis viruses, tuberculosis, brain cancer, and melanoma. Hypericum appears to hold substantial promise as a therapeutic agent for all of these illnesses. Nevertheless, considerably more research is called for, as clinical trials in humans have been limited and stringently controlled. People with any of these diseases should continue with conventional treatment protocols and only add hypericum as a supportive or adjunctive therapy under a doctor's advice.

• Use hypericum with caution, and only under the advice of a qualified practitioner, in children over the age of 12.

A Final Cautionary Endnote: The MAOI Controversy

When hypericum first came to medical and public attention as an effective antidepressant, early studies of its chemical properties strongly suggested that its therapeutic actions were most like those of a class of antidepressants called the monoamine oxidase inhibitors (MAOIs). The MAOIs, which include Nardil and Parnate, are very effective antidepressants, but they have a serious drawback. They can interact dangerously, and sometimes fatally, with foods and beverages that contain the amino acid tyramine and with other drugs or nutritional supplements that contain monoamines. Among other things, blood pressure can skyrocket to dangerous levels, threatening stroke and coma. People who take MAOIs for depression must therefore avoid a long list of foods, beverages, and medications.

Since hypericum was initially identified as an MAOI-like medication, people taking it were also cautioned to avoid the same foods and drugs as did those people taking prescription MAOIs.

Further research into hypericum's chemical properties, however, demonstrated that hypericum was much more like the selective serotonin reuptake inhibitors (SSRIs), of which Prozac is the most popular. The SSRIs do not interact with tyramine-containing substances. Therefore, the MAOI precautions were now considered not to apply to hypericum at all, though the herb continued to be erroneously identified in some popular literature as an MAOI. In fact, millions of German patients have been taking hypericum for years without having adverse MAOI-related reactions.

The latest research into hypericum's chemical properties seems to indicate that hypericum is in fact both an MAOI and an SSRI (and several other things as well!), but its MAOI properties are very mild and side effects appear to be mitigated when formulations use the whole plant.

At the time of this writing, it is generally believed that hypericum users do *not* have to avoid the same substances that MAOI users do, because its MAOI effect is mild. However, many practitioners prefer to err on the side of caution and routinely advise their patients who take hypericum to try to avoid, or restrict, certain foods, beverages, drugs, and nutritional supplements. We prefer to err on the side of caution as well, and below is an abbreviated list of those substances you should consider using with caution if you are taking hypericum.

- **Foods and Beverages to Use with Caution:** Wines and beers; aged or sharp cheeses; smoked or pickled meats and fishes; meat bouillons; sausages; powdered soups;

yeast and fava beans; soy sauce and soy products; yogurt and sour cream; tomatoes, eggplants, and avocados; raisins and bananas.

- **Drugs and Supplements to Use with Caution:** Cold, flu, and sinus remedies that contain nasal decongestants; diet pills; some hay fever and asthma medications; and amino acid supplements such as tyrosine.

❖

This in-depth focus on side effects, warnings, and precautions may appear to have the purpose of scaring you off hypericum. This isn't our intention! On the contrary, the clinical and practical information we have gathered about hypericum overwhelmingly points to its being remarkably safe and effective for a variety of illnesses and disorders.

In fact, among the small group of medicinal herbs currently receiving massive attention from conventional science—echinacea, ginkgo biloba, ginger, and kava, among others—hypericum has the best potential of being a "breakout" botanical. This may be the plant herb that effectively erases the divide of disbelief and skepticism that has existed for so long between alternative and conventional medicine.

If you follow the guidelines and precautions we have outlined in this chapter and work with a qualified medical practitioner as well, we heartily recommend that you try hypericum for any of the disorders we discuss in this book. To help you do just that, the next chapter describes how to find hypericum, how to buy it and use it, and even how to grow it!

CHAPTER 4

❖

Finding St. John's Wort
(Hypericum perforatum)

*The leaves, flowers, and seeds stamped, and put into a glass
with oyle olive, and set in the sunne for certain weeks together, and then strained ... doth make an oyle of the
colour of blood, which is a most precious remedy.*
—JOHN GERARD, SIXTEENTH-CENTURY BRITISH HERBALIST

Now that you have decided to try St. John's wort, how do
you go about finding it, buying it, and using it?

This chapter answers those questions and more. To begin
with, though—and especially if you are using St. John's wort
for the first time or have any chronic medical conditions—
we strongly recommend again that you seek the guidance of
a qualified medical practitioner. A holistic practitioner, one
who specializes in herbal or naturopathic medicine, may be
the best choice. And many holistic practitioners can provide
you with high-quality St. John's wort directly. The "Resources" section in the back of this book offers suggestions
on how to find a qualified alternative practitioner.

But don't discount your conventional (allopathic) physician either. Despite the bad press that many allopathic
physicians get from the alternative branch of medicine,
many general practitioners (GPs) and internists are well
aware of the benefits of St. John's wort—for depression
mostly—and are more than willing to work with their
patients who are looking for natural and safer alternatives to prescription medications. We know of one GP
in conservative southern New England who regularly

recommends St. John's wort to his mildly depressed patients and has had great success with it.

FINDING AND BUYING ST. JOHN'S WORT

Because St. John's wort has received such widespread attention and acclaim in the last two years, customer demand is great and finding a place that sells it is easier than ever. Keeping it in stock, however, may be a major problem for some smaller outlets, so shop around for a reliable and consistent supplier.

Most major drugstore chains, the pharmacy sections of large supermarket chains, and several large discount department store chains (such as Wal-Marts) now routinely stock St. John's wort—under its common name or as *Hypericum*—in tablet and capsule forms. Most health food stores carry St. John's wort in liquid extract, tablet, or capsule forms, and sometimes in dried herb form. You may also buy St. John's wort in any of its therapeutic forms—as well as hypericum seeds for growing the herb yourself—from a wealth of mail-order herbal suppliers by phone, fax, or e-mail. Our "Resources" section also provides a listing of some of the major suppliers of St. John's wort, together with phone and website information.

As we've mentioned above, St. John's wort comes in various forms—liquid extract, tablets, capsules, and dried herb—each of which has its pros and cons in terms of availability, therapeutic quality, and ease of use.

Buying High-Quality St. John's Wort

Quality, of course, is the number one issue and an increasingly critical one as inferior grades of St. John's wort are pushed into the marketplace to satisfy public demand. If you are going to use St. John's wort for depression, insomnia, SAD, or menstrual problems, to mention just a few of its medical indications, you want a formulation that is as therapeutically potent as possible, yet associated with the least side effects. Most practitioners therefore recommend that you use a hypericum formulation equivalent in potency to those used in the many successful clinical trials that studied the herb's effectiveness in treating depression.

Those clinical studies have taken place largely in Germany and Austria. There, the most commonly used hypericum formulation is Jarsin, also called LI 160, which is a gel capsule. (Other names used in Europe are Neuroplant and Psychotonin M.) These capsules contain 300 mg of hypericum that has been standardized to 0.3% of hypericin, the herb's most potent and active chemical constituent. The United States and Canada now have a variety of equivalent research-grade hypericum formulations available to the public through retail outlets and mail-order companies (see "Resources"). All are guaranteed as standardized to 0.3% hypericin and are marked accordingly on their labels. Do not buy a St. John's wort product that isn't marked as standardized.

Standardization simply means that the manufacturing process that converts a plant's parts into a herbal extract for consumption contains a checks-and-balances step, which ensures that a minimum percentage of one or more of the plant's most active chemical ingredients is always included in any batch. In the case of St. John's wort or hypericum, all herbal extract forms—liquid, tablets, capsules, or dried herb—should contain a minimum of 0.3% hypericin.

Let's take a brief look at the various forms in which St. John's wort is available, how each is generally manufactured and packaged, and their relative merits in terms of therapeutic potency and ease of use.

LIQUID EXTRACTS

Manufacturing and Packaging. Liquid herbal extracts (or tinctures) of St. John's wort are made by soaking chopped raw herb or crushed dried herb in alcohol (80% proof or more) or glycerine for two weeks in an airtight container that is shaken several times a day. The alcohol or glycerine extract and preserve the active chemical ingredients, while the inactive ingredients sink to the bottom of the container. At the end of the soaking period, the mixture is thoroughly strained. The liquid portion, containing the plant's active ingredients, is reserved and stored in tightly capped dark brown bottles that ensure the therapeutic potency of the herbal extract by protecting it from light. The caps of these bottles usually have a dropper built in for easy administration of the liquid.

The liquid medium in which a plant's herbs are soaked is called the *solvent* or *menstruum*, terms you may see on the label, along with the ratio of herb to liquid used in the manufacturing process. In alcohol extracts, a ratio of 1:1 is often standard and means that the dry weight of the herb equals the liquid volume of the solvent. For example, for every 1 pound or 16 *dry* ounces of fresh herb, 1 pint or 16 *liquid* ounces of alcohol are used as solvent.

Alcohol is the preferred solvent for liquid herbal extracts (some of the alcohol evaporates during the soaking process), because it best preserves the plant's active chemicals and extracts all the plant's constituents, including the volatile oils. Glycerine is also an excellent preservative and is an option for people who can't tolerate alcohol, but it doesn't extract all the plant's constituents. Some herbal extracts use apple-cider vinegar as a solvent, another nonalcoholic alternative.

The liquid extract method also is used to manufacture herbal oils, creams, and salves meant only for external use. For these formulations, rubbing alcohol is sometimes used as a solvent—and thus the preparations should never be taken internally. Olive and safflower oils are also popular solvents for herbs meant to be used topically.

Therapeutic Potency and Ease of Use. Liquid extracts generally are considered the preferred form in which to take medicinal herbs because they best preserve the plant's therapeutic chemical constituents. Both fresh and dried herbs can quickly lose their potency if they are not harvested and stored in optimal conditions before being made into tablets or capsules, or before being sold in bulk form (mostly to be used for teas).

Liquid extracts of plant herbs also have several other advantages over tablets, capsules, and dried herbs:

- Liquid extracts are the most highly concentrated forms of medicinal herbs and often less extract needs to be taken for therapeutic effect than an equivalent tablet or capsule form. This can be a cost savings in the long run, and may be gentler on the body as well.

- Liquid herbal extracts rapidly enter the bloodstream and thus their therapeutic effects are felt more quickly and efficiently.

- Liquid extracts retain their potency for a long time. Properly stored, they can be kept for up to ten years.

- Liquid extracts may be placed directly on or under the tongue for rapid absorption and are also readily diluted in water without losing potency.

   They also combine well with other herbs for making teas and combination herbal formulas.

- Adjusting the dosage of liquid extracts is often easier than with tablets or capsules, many of which can't effectively be cut in halves or thirds. For example, a common daily dosage of St. John's wort liquid extract is 20 to 30 drops (1/4 teaspoon to 1/2 teaspoon) three times a day, for a total of 60 to 90 drops a day. If you want to take St. John's wort in smaller doses more frequently throughout the day—perhaps to lessen side effects, as we discussed in Chapter 3—it is easy to adjust your dosage to 12 to 16 drops, five times a day.

There are disadvantages to liquid herbal extracts as well.

- One, they are initially more expensive than tablet or capsule forms (but sometimes more economical over the long run).

- Two, liquid extracts may come in a wide variety of potencies, due to the solvent used or the ratio of herb to solvent employed, and thus the range of recommended drops per day may run from as low as 60 (for standard therapeutic potencies) to as high as 200 (for lower potency extracts).
    Our discussion here, for example, centers on liquid extracts or tinctures that use alcohol or glycerine in a herb-to-liquid ratio of 1:1. A standard daily dose would be 60 drops. Extracts with ratios of 1:1 have the greater therapeutic potency but may carry the risk of more intense side effects, such as stomach upset. On the other hand, liquid extracts with ratios of 1:5—where there is far more liquid than fresh herbs— usually have less therapeutic potency because active ingredients are more diluted. These formulations require you to take higher daily doses to get the desired

therapeutic effect. Follow the manufacturer's instructions on the extract's label, but err on the side of caution when a range of drops is given. Start out with the lowest dose possible, gradually increasing your dosage as necessary.

• Another sometimes distinct disadvantage of liquid extracts is that their taste and odor are far more intense than in tablet or capsule forms—and many plant herbs have a decidedly noxious taste and smell. Fortunately, St. John's wort is not one of the more unpleasant-tasting or -smelling of the medicinal herbs, and diluting it in spring water makes it even more palatable.

• Finally, the best liquid herbal extracts are those that are extracted with alcohol, which many people can't or won't take. Glycerine is a fine alternative, but you may lose some therapeutic potency.

TABLETS AND CAPSULES
Manufacturing and Packaging. The rendering of plant herbs into tablets and capsules has grown increasingly more sophisticated, and these forms of St. John's wort often rival the therapeutic potency of liquid extract.

Tablets and capsules are comprised of the dried plant herb that has been ground to a fine powder. Of course, a high-quality tablet or capsule is only as good as the purity, freshness, and potency of the raw plant herb from which the powder is made. Both freshly picked and dried medicinal plants lose their therapeutic potency quickly if not grown, harvested, and stored properly.

Many herbal books offer wonderful instructions for making your own tablets and capsules from raw bulk herb, but we don't recommend it unless you are 100 percent sure that the supplier is providing fresh and potent herb. Instead, we recommend that you buy tablets and capsules that are premanufactured by a reputable herbal supplier.

Tablets, which are somewhat less popular than capsules, are manufactured by means of a complex commercial process that involves grinding the dried herb into fine powder, mixing it with a binder (such as guar gum) to hold the formulation together, adding a water-based substance that allows the pill to break down easily in the body when taken with water, and, finally, coating the pill with a lubricant such as vegetable oil, which allows for easy swallowing. Tablets may vary greatly in size, from quite tiny to very large, depending on the herb and quantity used. Tablets usually contain more herb than do capsules and tend to retain the original "taste" of the plant herb—an advantage or disadvantage, depending on the herb.

Capsules are a more popular form of herbal medicine and easier to make than tablets. The dried herb is finely ground into a powder, and the powder is then added to preformed gelatin capsules. Both vegetable and animal gelatin capsules are available. Capsules, too, vary greatly in size; some are so large that many people find them difficult to swallow. On the other hand, a good many other people tolerate capsules better than tablets, and capsules have the additional advantage of masking the unpleasant taste of some herbs.

Therapeutic Potency and Ease of Use. Although liquid extracts generally are preferred by practitioners, tablets and capsules are very popular among consumers. They are often therapeutically equivalent to the liquid form, and have several advantages over some of the liquid extracts:

- Because there is no straining process in the making of herbal powders, both tablets and capsules may contain more of the whole plant and thus more of *all* its active chemical constituents. For example, liquid extracts that use glycerine as the solvent cannot extract a plant's volatile oils, and many plants' most active chemical constituents are found in the volatile oils. This is not a critical issue in the case of St. John's wort, since several of its most active chemical constituents (hypericin and hyperforin among them) are found throughout the plant.

  Nevertheless, traditional herbalists are also adamant about the fact that all parts of a plant work together synergistically, balancing and supporting one another in the healing process. Thus, traditional practitioners believe that the full therapeutic effect of a plant herb is experienced only when the *whole* plant is used in a formulation.

- Tablets and capsules are easy and convenient to use and store.

- They are easy to find and buy and sometimes less expensive than liquid extracts.

- Tablets and capsules don't contain alcohol.

- Some tablets and most capsules tend to mask the unpleasant taste and smell of some herbs far better than do liquid extracts, though this isn't a big consideration with St. John's wort, which is relatively benign in taste and smell. (Interestingly, traditional herbalists would consider this particular "advantage" of tablets and capsules a disadvantage instead, since the taste of some herbs, particularly the very bitter ones, are considered crucial to the therapeutic process.)

• In the case of St. John's wort specifically, capsules and tablets containing the dried plant's powder were used in most of the successful clinical studies we describe in this book, so we know they work well. Commercially available tablets and capsules also come in the same form and dosage as those used in research studies— 300 mg each, standardized to 0.3% hypericin.

Tablets and capsules have several disadvantages too:

• They may be difficult to swallow or digest.

• Capsules tend to lose their potency fairly quickly, some within three to twelve months. (Tablets retain their potency longer.) Capsules also may contain less plant herb than do tablets and liquid extracts.

• The single greatest disadvantage of tablets and capsules is that they are more vulnerable to tampering and adulteration by unscrupulous or careless manufacturers. Inferior grades of a plant herb, nontherapeutic plant substances, and even nonplant substances may be easily added to powdered herbs as filler or to increase dry weight. This could become a serious problem in the case of St. John's wort. Demand is rapidly exceeding supply, and some suppliers may be tempted to cut corners by using filler. Always check to see that your St. John's wort is provided by a reputable supplier, particularly when you are buying tablets or capsules. (Our "Resources" section may help you find a reliable manufacturer or distributor.)

BULK DRIED HERB

Manufacturing and Packaging. Bulk dried herb is available from many traditional herbal shops, from neighborhood herbalists, from herbal medical practitioners, and from some manufacturers and distributors.

The medicinal plant is usually harvested right after its active growing season and just before the plant is in full flower. This is the time when the plant's active chemical constituents are most potent. The blossoms, buds, stems, and leaves of healthy plants are gently cut and gathered, then spread out to dry naturally, sometimes for several weeks. They are carefully monitored and turned for even drying. Since plant herbs can lose their therapeutic potency very quickly after harvesting, they must be dried and stored under rigorous care.

After plant herbs are thoroughly dried, they may be prepared for shipping or selling in one of several ways: as the whole plant (including leaves, flowers, buds, seeds, and roots—if applicable); cut up into small pieces and sifted to remove twigs, thorns, and other hard matter; sliced (when the root only is used, as in burdock and licorice); or powdered.

Dried herbs are commonly shipped and sold in large bins or storage jars. In fact, shops usually leave them in these containers for display; you can buy them by weight and take them home in small plastic bags.

Most dried herb is bought after it's already been cut up into small pieces. This makes it easier to prepare the herb at home, usually as teas (or what herbalists call an *infusion*). We don't recommend using a St. John's wort tea for treating a condition such as depression; a tea is simply not potent enough for that indication. However, St. John's wort tea can be a wonderful therapeutic aid for anxiety, insomnia, colds, and flus, as well as some of the symptoms of PMS or menstrual and menopausal problems. It is also an effective weight loss aid. At the end of this section, we give you directions for making your own St. John's Wort tea from dried and cut-up herb, together with some suggestions for other plant herbs that combine wonderfully with St. John's wort.

Therapeutic Potency and Ease of Use. For St. John's wort in particular, the dried herb form is considered the least therapeutically potent. We agree with this for a condition such as depression. But the dried herb prepared as a tea can be a powerful healing tool for other medical problems, as we mentioned above. In fact, dried herbs prepared as teas, infusions, and decoctions (a method similar to an infusion, but used with root herbs or woody herbs that require a longer cooking time) has been the preferred treatment method in Chinese herbal medicine for several millennia. There are other advantages to using dried herbs.

- Despite what you may read in some books, properly harvested, dried, and stored herbs retain much of their potency for up to a year. They must, of course, be carefully stored and regularly checked for deterioration.

- Dried herbs have the additional advantage of retaining all the active chemical constituents of the plant in their purest and most natural forms. We know from the latest clinical research published about St. John's wort that the whole plant seems to have more therapeutic potential than do several of its active constituents when they are isolated and synthesized.

- Dried herbs lend themselves to a variety of uses, beyond being made into teas, infusions, and decoctions for internal use:

—A handful of dried St. John's wort may be added to a healing footbath that not only soothes aching feet, but also may help fight an oncoming cold!

—Several ounces of dried St. John's wort may be wrapped in cheesecloth or muslin and added to bathwater for an anxiety-relieving and sleep-promoting soak.

—If you are really ambitious, you can even make your own St. John's wort capsules at home from dried herb. The preformed gelatin capsules are available in a variety of sizes from health food stores and other suppliers of natural food products. Use your blender at high speed to grind the dried herb into a fine powder. Spread the powder on a plate or tray, pull apart a capsule, and scoop the powder into both ends. Reseal the two halves and you have your own homemade medication—quality assured!

Dried herb also has several disadvantages:

• Dried herb may be difficult to find and its quality hard to assess.

• Even properly stored dried herb will lose its potency in a year. And of all the herb forms, dried herb is the most susceptible to infestation and environmental degradation.

• Dried herb does not have the convenience and ease of use that liquid extracts, tablets, and capsules do. Preparation time is required to use dried herb in any of its therapeutic forms.

St. John's Wort Tea

❖

Use 1 teaspoon of dried St. John's wort—or 3 teaspoons of fresh herb—for each 8-ounce cup of tea you are going to brew. Place the dried or fresh herb in a glass or enameled teapot that you have prewarmed with some hot water. Pour boiling water over the dried or fresh herbs, cover the pot, and allow the tea to steep for 15 minutes. After the tea has steeped, pour into individual mugs, using a small kitchen strainer to catch the tea grounds. Flavor your tea with honey, licorice root, or brown sugar.

For medicinal purposes, drink St. John's wort tea at least three times a day.

Some of the other herbs that blend wonderfully with St. John's wort in tea include balm *(Melissa officinalis)*, echinacea *(Echinacea augustifolia)*, passionflower *(Passiflora incarnata)*, rosehips *(Rosa canina)*, and valerian *(Valeriana officinalis)*. To make a combination herbal tea, combine equal parts of 1 teaspoon or more of each herb and boil 8 ounces of water for every teaspoon used. (For fresh herbs, use three times the quantity of dried herbs.) Steep and flavor as for St. John's Wort tea.

A FINAL NOTE ON BUYING AND USING ST. JOHN'S WORT

The Whole Plant vs. Its Parts

When you buy St. John's wort, in liquid extract, tablet, or capsule forms, the package label may claim that the herb was processed only from the flowers and/or buds of the plant. In the absence of such a claim, the herb was most likely processed from the whole plant, including flowers, buds, leaves, and stems. Which is better? To date, there is no clear answer.

Seminal research into hypericum's therapeutic potential for treating depression identified hypericin, the plant's most active chemical constituent, as solely responsible for hypericum's antidepressant effects. Hypericin is found throughout the plant, but occurs in greatest concentrations in the unopened buds and in the flowers. Since hypericum has been primarily used for depression, formulations prepared from the buds and flowers of St. John's wort were considered the most therapeutically powerful and therefore preferable to products made from the whole plant. Additionally, the groundbreaking research conducted at New York University Medical Center in the late 1980s into hypericum's potent anti-AIDS and other antiviral properties has used a synthetic form of hypericin.

The most current pharmacological research into hypericum's properties, however, indicates that its potent therapeutic constituents are found *throughout* the plant. In fact, hypericin is no longer considered solely responsible for hypericum's antidepressant properties.

Our recommendation? Formulations of St. John's wort made from the whole plant are probably just as effective as those made from buds and flowers only, and in fact may even be a little better because they retain the synergistic therapeutic action of all the plant's constituents. If whole-plant formulations are more readily available and less costly for you, we see no reason not to use them.

On the other hand, if you are planning to use St. John's wort strictly for depression or its antiviral properties, and you prefer to take the cautious route, by all means buy a St. John's wort formulation made from buds and flowers only.

❖

GROWING YOUR OWN ST. JOHN'S WORT

For the ambitious, the adventurous, and the ardent gardeners among you, growing St. John's wort is surprisingly easy and immensely rewarding. The bright yellow flowers are a delightful harbinger of summer, and both harvesting and drying the plant are simple and fun. In addition, the process of planting, cultivating, and preparing your own herbs is wonderfully therapeutic in itself.

We do, however, recommend only using your home-grown St. John's wort in healing teas as short-term or supportive therapy. For clinical indications, such as depression, where specific dosage and therapeutic strength is critical to successful treatment, buying high-quality manufactured hypericum is the better route to go. If you do want to grow your own St. John's wort, here are the basics.

Planting St. John's Wort

You may buy St. John's wort seeds, seedlings, or small starter plants at many plant nurseries and herb farms. Our "Resources" section also lists mail-order plant and seed providers.

You will need a patch of open land in your yard or garden that's at least 3 feet by 3 feet. The area should be sunny, have good drainage, and receive plenty of circulating air. Above all, the soil should *not* be prepared before sowing or planting. In fact, St. John's wort thrives in poor, even damaged and calcified, soil. It also grows in partial shade, if unavoidable.

Follow the directions on the seed package (or the instructions that come with starter plants) for sowing St. John's wort. Depending on where you live, plant St. John's wort in the fall or spring. Sow starter plants at a depth of about 5 inches. Sow seeds shallowly, just beneath the soil, about 5 inches apart. Water sparingly and never fertilize or prune the plants. Of course, you never want to use pesticides on your plants either.

If you have particularly cold winters in your area, cover your plantings with a protective sheet at night during the coldest and snowiest part of the season, but always give them about five hours of full sunlight during the day.

St. John's wort grows to a height of 4 to 6 inches during the first year, begins budding in the second year, and achieves its full height (from 1 to 3 feet) by the third year. A perennial plant, St. John's wort dies back in the winter, but reseeds itself in the early spring.

You can plant St. John's wort by itself or in a formal herb garden—as long as it has enough room to spread its roots. Other herb plants that grow well with St. John's wort include dandelion, raspberry, peppermint, and goldenrod. Allow about 3 square feet between herb plants, so they have room to grow and you have room to harvest.

HARVESTING AND DRYING ST. JOHN'S WORT

Harvesting. In the northern hemisphere, St. John's wort is generally harvested from summer through fall. Summer harvesting begins right after the plant's most active growing season in the spring (sometime in early to mid-June) just before the plant flowers. This is the time when the potent buds and early, young flowers are harvested. Harvesting often continues through August or as long as the plant flowers. You may want to harvest buds and early flowers in June, and then periodically harvest buds, flowers, leaves, and stems throughout the remainder of the growing season.

Choose a dry, sunny, moderately warm day to begin harvesting. Use sharp garden scissors or a knife to gently cut healthy buds, flowers, and leaves that are free from insect bites, weather spots, or withering.

Drying. Choose a warm, sunny, well-ventilated and protected spot on your porch or in a kitchen window to dry the plant. First cut the leaves, flowers, and buds from the stem of the plant. Then lay out all the cut parts of the plant, including stems, in single layers on racks. Oven racks and baker's cooling racks are perfect for this step. Drying times will vary, depending on the age of the plant and weather conditions. Generally, from ten days to two weeks is needed for the plant parts to dry to the point where they are brittle and easily crumbled. During this time, turn the plant parts once or twice a day to ensure even drying.

When the plant parts are dried, immediately store them in a dry, nonporous container with a tight-fitting lid. A metal, ceramic, or dark-glass canister is the best choice. Do not use plastic containers, since they may absorb some of the plant's medicinal oils. Store the canister in a dry area away from direct heat and sunlight. Use as needed, and enjoy!

❖

Now it's time to move on to Part II of our book, about using St. John's wort to treat specific illnesses and conditions.

Part I has been designed to teach you the basics about St. John's wort: its long and illustrious history; its astonishing and wide-ranging therapeutic actions for a variety of illnesses; the advantages and the drawbacks of using St. John's wort; and finally, how to buy it, take it, and even grow it. Still, the most exciting information is yet to come: how St. John's wort may help you to effectively, naturally, and gently treat body, mind, and soul.

PART II

❖

Putting St. John's Wort
to Work for You

Using St. John's Wort to Treat Body, Mind, and Spirit

Part II of this book discusses how to use St. John's wort (hypericum) for a variety of illnesses and medical conditions, including mild-to-moderate depression, seasonal affective disorder (SAD), premenstrual syndrome (PMS), menstrual problems, menopausal symptoms, insomnia, cold and flu viruses, and lowered immunity. We also discuss its use as an aid to weight loss.

We briefly describe each illness or condition and review the conventional medical treatments for them. Then we describe how St. John's wort may be used as an alternative treatment. We do this with a view toward both the traditional therapeutic uses of St. John's wort and the latest scientific research that confirms its therapeutic properties.

We describe how St. John's wort may work to treat specific symptoms of the illness or condition, followed by appropriate suggestions about what form of the herb to take (liquid, capsules, or dried herb in the form of tea, for example), what dosage to take and at what times, and how long treatment should last. Wherever appropriate, we also offer suggestions for other practical and alternative treatments that may be helpful, including herbs that work well in combination with St. John's wort.

Interspersed throughout this section are more personal stories of everyday people who have used St. John's wort with great success for a variety of conditions. Their names and occupations have been changed, but their stories are true.

We have based our recommendations for how to use St. John's wort, including dosages and treatment length, in part on our knowledge of how St. John's wort has been used traditionally by herbal medical practitioners for centuries and also on our own knowledge of herbal medicine in general. We also based our therapeutic recommendations on the extensive clinical research published in the last ten years about hypericum's effectiveness in treating depression.

The treatment of depression, in fact, serves as an excellent model for reliably extending the therapeutic use of St. John's wort to the other medical conditions covered in this book. As the following chapter amply illustrates, clinical depression involves a complex mix of physical and mental symptoms, including mood swings, eating disorders, insomnia and other sleep disturbances, fatigue, headaches, vague aches and pain, general physical debilitation, and greater susceptibility to viral and bacterial infections. Substantial clinical research in depressed patients indicates that St. John's wort may successfully target and treat *all* these varying symptoms. Thus it clearly has enormous therapeutic potential as a wide-ranging, one-of-a-kind medical treatment.

As enthusiastic and confident as we are about St. John's wort, we also cannot stress enough how important we believe it is that you work with a qualified medical practitioner—alternative or conventional—if you take St. John's wort even on a short-term basis. The enormous therapeutic potential and scientifically confirmed properties of St. John's wort may appear to be the stuff of miracles, but St. John's wort is no New Age panacea and this book is not meant to suggest that. On the contrary.

Depression, for example, is a very serious illness. It requires a thorough diagnosis, a meticulous and encompassing treatment plan, and careful monitoring by you and your practitioner. Chronic and debilitating menstrual pain, to use another example, may be a symptom of a more serious underlying medical condition that may require surgery. Repeated viral and bacterial infections may be a red flag that something is terribly amiss in the body's immune system. A qualified medical practitioner can rule out such serious medical complications. You also may not be able to use St. John's wort if you have certain chronic medical conditions, or are taking certain medications. Finally, St. John's wort may just not work for you.

With that in mind, we hope you enjoy learning how to use St. John's wort as a safe, natural, and effective alternative to conventional drugs.

CHAPTER 5

❖

Treating Depression
with St. John's Wort

*In a 4-week treatment study, 900 mg of hypericum [daily]
was associated with a significant reduction in the total
score of the Hamilton Depression Rating Scale. Overall,
hypericum was well tolerated and therefore the data suggest that pharmacological treatment with hypericum may
be an efficient therapy in patients with SAD [seasonal
affective disorder].*
—PHARMACOPSYCHIATRY SEPTEMBER 30, 1997

The American Psychiatric Association (APA) estimates
that about 1 in 4 women and 1 in 10 men will experience a
significant depression in their lifetime. In fact, in any given
year in the United States, an estimated 18 million people
suffer from depression and more than half of them never
receive treatment. Among those people who are most
seriously depressed, more than 30,000 will take their own
lives. Depression, the most common of mental illnesses
and a serious medical condition that takes an enormous
toll on personal and professional lives, is notoriously
underdiagnosed and undertreated. One reason for this is
the social stigma still attached to mental illness. Another
equally insidious reason is the fact that depression simply
goes unrecognized. In an increasingly chaotic, fragmented,
and high-stress world, many of the symptoms of depression masquerade as "normal" conditions of late-twentieth-
century life.

Recognizing depression, therefore, is the first step
toward treatment.

RECOGNIZING DEPRESSION

All of us have times in our lives when we feel sad, confused, anxious, angry, lonely, and lost. These are normal reactions to the grief and madness contemporary life throws our way. Death, illness, loss, betrayal, separation, poverty, aging, violence—these are just some of the things that suddenly may turn our lives upside down. Faced with any of these challenges, it is natural for us to turn away from the world for a while, take time to regather our strength and our spirit, and then learn how to carry on. Slowly we begin to enjoy life anew, to take pleasure in our families and friends, and to look forward to the future.

When we cannot shake off life's indignities, when day after day rolls by wrapped in a dark cloud, when seemingly nothing brings us pleasure or solace, we have moved from simple sadness and grief to the state of depression. And we need help.

Defining Depression

Depression is a serious mental illness. Most medical practitioners define it as a mental state characterized by an inability to derive any pleasure or happiness from the simple things in life—spouses and lovers, children, friends, sex, food, work, music, or nature. And while it's normal to have a day or two when nothing makes us happy, the inability to enjoy life for a prolonged period of time is not normal. It is a red flag that something has gone terribly wrong inside us.

Still, we often excuse or ignore this key marker for depression because it may masquerade as one or more of a constellation of symptoms, many of which we accept as normal in our hectic world: no appetite, no energy, no interest in anyone or anything; sadness, sleep difficulties, confusion and foggy thinking, anger and irritability, vague aches and pains that never go away, seeking solace in drugs, alcohol, and sex, and at the darkest end of the spectrum, recurrent thoughts of death and suicide. These are all recognized medical symptoms of depression.

As for what causes depression to begin with, most research seems to indicate that the causes are a complex blend of psychosocial influences (what happens to us and what we learn as children and adults), biochemical responses (how our bodies and brains respond to what happens in our lives), and genetic predisposition (whether depression runs in our families). The fact that there may not be any one cause or reason for depression can make diagnosis and treatment difficult and long-term.

For some of us, the symptoms of depression begin as natural reactions to a life-changing event or unpleasant incident. But instead of going away with time, they become ingrained in the very fabric of who we are and how we view the world. For others of us, living with these symptoms is a lifelong challenge that may start as early as childhood. The number of symptoms we have, how intensely we experience them, and how long they have lasted all determine a diagnosis of depression.

---------------------- ❖ ----------------------

Lyla's Story:
Combating Depression the Natural Way

Lyla, a secretary in the garment industry in New York, began to experience some symptoms of severe depression in her late twenties, not long after she lost her mother to breast cancer. There was no history of clinical depression in Lyla's family, and her bouts with depression seemed to be intermittent and not chronic.

"About two years ago I began having spells of deep, deep depression. I would have crying jags just about every day—anything could set me off—and sometimes this would happen in the most inappropriate places, like at work or in a supermarket. I would become overwhelmed with feelings of loss and isolation and loneliness and fear. And then I would just lose it, wherever I was. I had always been pretty health conscious before this started happening, but now I began either skipping meals entirely or bingeing late at night. And I stopped exercising. I wasn't having trouble sleeping though. If anything, I slept way too much. I'd nap in the afternoon, after work, and stay up late at night. Then I'd sleep like the dead through my alarm the next morning, only to wake up in a panic, knowing I'd be late for work. The funny thing was, at first this would go on for a week or two and then just stop. I'd seem to snap out of it for a while, then a month or so later the cycle would start up again. I knew some of this had to do with watching my mother die, and losing her, and I thought it would go away after time, after I had gotten all the grief out of me.

"But then these cycles began to get closer and closer together, and my moods got darker and darker. My performance on the job was suffering, and I was alienating my friends, who couldn't stand to be around me anymore. Frankly, I couldn't blame them. Then about fourteen months ago, during one of these 'spells,' I began to think about suicide. Seriously. And that frightened me a lot. I called my best friend, and she begged me to get professional help. I did. I began sessions with a wonderful therapist, whom I saw twice a week. She also prescribed Prozac for me, which I took for about three months. But I hated it. It made me feel jumpy and weird, and I asked to be taken off it. I really didn't want to take any drugs at all. I thought therapy should be enough. But my doctor disagreed. I wasn't thinking about suicide anymore, but I still had a lot of dark moods and physically I was very drained. In fact, I had asked for, and gotten, a six-month leave of absence from work. My doctor felt I still needed some kind of medication.

"She had been reading a good deal about St. John's wort, and she asked me if I would give it a try. I agreed, and I started using it as soon as I was weaned off the Prozac. I took the liquid extract, about twenty drops in a glass of water, three times a day. I have to say it took about four or five weeks before I noticed any changes, but when I did notice them, they were incredible. Those dark moods just seemed to lift, and I felt calmer and more centered. I had never had trouble sleeping, but now my sleep seemed deeper and more restful. This was just in the first couple of months. After almost a year on St. John's wort, I have to say I feel one hundred percent better—make that one thousand percent better! And I haven't noticed any adverse effects at all.

"I'm back at work, and I also just went back to school at night for my B.A. I still see the same therapist, but once a week now. She's been incredible. Depression is nothing to mess with. And I expect to stay on St. John's wort for at least another year. It's worked incredibly for me."

❖

Diagnosing Depression

The American Psychiatric Association and the National Institutes of Health (NIH) have issued guidelines for diagnosing depression, also called **mood disorder** or **clinical depression**. Among the major symptoms they list are:

- feeling sad or depressed for most of the day

- loss of appetite, overeating, or other eating disorders, including sudden weight loss or weight gain

- feelings of guilt, worthlessness, or hopelessness

- sleep difficulties, including insomnia, inability to stay asleep through the night, or oversleeping

- inability to concentrate, slowness in thought, loss of energy, general fatigue

- loss of interest or pleasure in everyday activities

- vague or chronic body aches and pains that appear to have no physical origin and don't respond to standard treatment

- irritability and agitation

- recurrent thoughts of death or suicide, or attempted suicide

Furthermore, there are four basic types of depression, each one distinguished from the other by the nature and number of the above symptoms that are present, the severity or intensity of those symptoms, and how long they have been present.

The four major types of depression are: **major depressive disorder, dysthymic disorder, bipolar disorder** (manic-depression), and **cyclothymic disorder.** Let's look briefly at each one.

- **Major Depressive Disorder.** According to the APA and NIH diagnostic guidelines, a diagnosis of major depressive disorder (major depression) should be considered—and a thorough medical evaluation conducted—if a person has four or more of the above symptoms nearly every day for more than two weeks, or to such a degree that they significantly affect family, work, and other areas of the person's life. Additionally, one of the symptoms experienced *must* be either sadness or depression for most of the day, *or* loss of interest/pleasure in everyday activities.

  Major depressive disorder is the most commonly diagnosed depression and is characterized as mild, moderate, or severe, depending on the number and intensity of the symptoms. The majority of major depressive disorders fall into the mild-to-moderate range and 80 percent of these are fully treatable.

  There are also several subgroups of major depressions, including the **postpartum depression** experienced by many women during the first weeks or months after childbirth, and **seasonal affective disorder (SAD),** the depression seasonally triggered during autumn and winter that appears to be related to diminishing sunlight.

- **Dysthymic Disorder.** With dysthymic depression, a person experiences a number of the classic symptoms of depression but at a much lower intensity than in a major depressive disorder. However, this "low level" functioning form of depression is present almost all the time, every day, over a very long period of time—a minimum of two years. In fact, many dysthymic depressions begin in childhood and continue throughout a person's life. Later in life, they often progress to a major depression, and when that happens, a person is diagnosed with having "double depression."

- **Bipolar Disorder.** Also known as manic-depression, bipolar disorder is chiefly characterized by alternating periods of extreme emotional highs (mania) and severe emotional lows (major depression). Bipolar depression appears to have a clearly biochemical and/or genetic basis. It is a far less common type of depression, affecting only about 1 percent of the population, and it often requires lifelong medication—lithium is usually the drug of choice—as well as careful medical supervision.

- **Cyclothymic Disorder.** Similar to dysthymic depression's relationship to major depression, cyclothymic disorder is a milder form of bipolar disorder. A person with cyclothymic disorder also experiences alternating periods of emotional highs and lows, but at a far less intense level than in classic manic-depression. Also like dysthymia, cyclothymic depressions may begin in childhood or young adulthood and frequently progress to bipolar disorders.

❖

It's important to note here that the extensive body of research confirming the effectiveness of St. John's wort in treating depression has focused exclusively on treating mild-to-moderate forms of major depression, dysthymic depression, and SAD. Before we discuss the use of St. John's wort as an alternative treatment for those types of depression, we should look at some of the conventional forms of treating depression.

CONVENTIONAL TREATMENTS FOR DEPRESSION

Conventional medicine traditionally has treated depression with psychotherapy, antidepressant drugs, or a combination of both. For many mild to moderate forms of depression, particularly those that are "reactive" in nature—that is, those that arise in response to a life-changing event— psychotherapy alone may be sufficient. When psychotherapy alone isn't enough, a treatment plan combining therapy and antidepressant drugs is often the next best course. Far too frequently, however, antidepressant drugs are prescribed alone, often by a family physician, without the crucial backup of at least some initial psychotherapy. Since all depressions have both a psychosocial and a biochemical component, both modes of treatment are usually needed.

Let's take a look at the psychotherapeutic approach first.

Using Psychotherapy to Treat Depression

Psychotherapy, or what is commonly called "talk" therapy, focuses on the verbal and emotional interaction between a trained therapist and a patient. Through mutual talking and listening, the patient and the therapist work together to help reframe the patient's view of, and response to, the world. Patients are guided toward creating better coping mechanisms, finding workable solutions to their specific problems, and repairing or strengthening their personal relationships.

Three basic forms of psychotherapy are used to treat depression: cognitive therapy, behavioral therapy, and interpersonal therapy.

- **Cognitive therapy** focuses on helping patients change their negative or depressive views and thoughts about the world and about specific social situations.

- **Behavioral therapy** focuses on helping patients transform negative or self-defeating behaviors into positive and self-affirming behaviors.

- **Interpersonal therapy** focuses on helping patients improve their personal relationships.

Most psychotherapy for depression is short-term, lasting usually no more than twenty visits of an hour each, and improvement is usually felt in two to three months. When therapy sessions aren't enough to ease the symptoms of depression, or when symptoms are more severe, antidepressant drugs are frequently prescribed as an adjunct to psychotherapy.

Using Antidepressant Drugs to Treat Depression

Antidepressant drugs have revolutionized the treatment of depression because they so effectively and dramatically relieve or stabilize many of the physical and emotional symptoms of depression. And when depressed persons feel better physically and emotionally, they are also better equipped to make the psychosocial changes necessary to alleviate their depression.

The symptoms of depression are in part caused by complex biochemical changes or imbalances in the brain's chemistry. Biochemicals called neurotransmitters are responsible for harmoniously processing the billions of chemical "messages" that the brain transmits throughout the body from moment to moment. Many of these chemical messages concern emotions, memories, stress responses, general well-being, pleasure, and pain.

Three key neurotransmitters have been associated with the symptoms of depression. They are serotonin, which is associated with a general sense of well-being; dopamine, which is directly responsible for pleasurable feelings; and norepinephrine, which affects mental alertness and physical energy.

When these neurotransmitters are functioning well and are at optimal levels in the brain, we experience a sense of happiness, well-being, security, balance, clear thinking, and boundless energy. But when the neurotransmitters malfunction, or their levels significantly drop or rise, our thoughts, emotions, sense of well-being, and even physical health are affected in turn.

Antidepressants are designed both to restore equilibrium to the neurotransmitter system and to act directly on the biochemicals responsible for feelings of depression, pleasure, and well-being.

Three major groups of antidepressants have been used over the last thirty years. They are the monoamine oxidase inhibitors (MAOIs), the tricyclic antidepressants (TCAs), and the selective serotonin reuptake inhibitors (SSRIs). All the antidepressants are slow-acting drugs and must be taken for several weeks before their effect is appreciably felt. Let's take a look at how each class of antidepressant works in the brain.

- **MAOIs.** This group of antidepressant drugs increases the levels of serotonin in the brain by suppressing (inhibiting) an enzyme called monoamine oxidase. Monoamine oxidase breaks down serotonin and thus decreases the quantity of serotonin available in the brain. Serotonin is a powerful neurotransmitter responsible for general feelings of physical and mental well-being and emotional stability. Normal levels of serotonin contribute to our feeling good, but low levels can cause anxiousness, anger, irritability, and a generally depressed feeling. By inhibiting the action of monoamine oxidase on serotonin, the MAOIs in effect raise serotonin levels and the pleasurable feelings that go along with them.

Examples of popular MAOIs are Nardil (phenelzine) and Parnate (tranylcypromine), both of which are quite effective in treating depression. But the MAOIs, like all prescription antidepressants, have bothersome and sometimes serious side effects and aren't tolerated well by some individuals. The major drawback of the MAOIs, however, is how they interact with certain foods, beverages, and prescription and over-the-counter drugs that contain the enzyme tyramine. Examples of tyramine-containing substances include aged cheeses, red wines, soy sauce, salami, some cold medications, and some antibiotics. When combined with any of the tyramine-containing substances, MAOIs can produce dangerous and potentially life-threatening reactions. These include a sudden rise in blood pressure, chest pain, nausea, and possible stroke. Because people taking MAOIs must avoid a significant number of foods, drinks, and medications, these antidepressants are now less frequently prescribed.

• TCAs. The tricyclic antidepressants, named for the unique three-ring structure of their chemical composition, are a first-generation group of antidepressants that date back to the 1950s and that were very popular in the seventies and eighties. The TCAs work directly to increase the levels of the neurotransmitters epinephrine, norepinephrine, and dopamine—also called catecholamines. Norepinephrine and dopamine are critically involved in regulating both the central nervous system and the cardiovascular system.

Some well-known TCAs include Elavil (amitriptyline), Sinequan (doxepin), and imipramine (Tofranil). Considered the "gold standard" of antidepressants, imipramine is the one against which the effectiveness of other antidepressants, including St. John's wort, has been tested. The TCAs are remarkably effective in treating depressions, particularly those that involve weight loss, depressed moods, and the inability to experience pleasure. But the TCAs also have been associated with some serious side effects, including sexual dysfunction, confusion, blurred vision, sluggishness, low blood pressure, rapid heartbeat, and, very rarely, seizures. Further, they are not recommended for people with cardiac and urinary tract problems, and this proviso excludes many older patients.

- **SSRIs.** The selective serotonin reuptake inhibitors are the newest and most popular class of antidepressants. They block the natural reuptake (absorption) of serotonin into brain cells and thus keep the levels of circulating serotonin high. The SSRIs appear to be better tolerated than the other groups of antidepressants, though they can cause insomnia, jitteriness, impotence, dry mouth, and diarrhea. The SSRIs also must be used cautiously with older people or those with kidney or liver problems.

Two popular SSRIs are Prozac (fluoxetine) and

Zoloft (sertraline), with Prozac by far the most popular and most prescribed of the two. It is also prescribed for obsessive-compulsive disorder and bulimia, particularly when they are associated with symptoms of depression.

Prozac appears to have somewhat less intense side effects than the other antidepressants, but it remains in the body for a long time after a person stops using it. Therefore, caution must be taken when switching from Prozac to another serotonin-based antidepressant. And many people do in fact stop taking Prozac. It doesn't work for all depressions, and some of its side effects are disturbing, including possible rapid weight loss and insomnia. These same people are often subsequently prescribed an MAOI, but the combination of the two antidepressants can cause a potentially fatal condition called **serotonin syndrome**. With serotonin syndrome, too much serotonin floods the body, causing agitation, tremors, muscle spasms, abrupt changes in blood pressure, and sometimes coma.

Drug manufacturers caution physicians and patients alike to wait at least five weeks after stopping Prozac before taking another serotonin-based antidepressant such as an MAOI. Alternatively, people stopping an MAOI should wait at least two weeks before taking Prozac.

All antidepressants were originally formulated to be taken on a short-term basis—one year at the most—and as an adjunct to psychotherapy. Many people, however, take antidepressants for much longer periods of time, even over the course of a lifetime. This is often not necessary for mild-to-moderate depressions. And as with all prescribed medications, long-term use of synthetic drugs also raises the spectre of increased and more serious side effects as people get older. Antidepressant drugs are expensive too, some costing from $200 to $300 a month for a daily regimen.

That's why the news of a natural antidepressant like St. John's wort has met with such enthusiasm and generated a wealth of research. It is comparable in effect to Prozac, perhaps more effective than imipramine, is far less expensive than prescription antidepressants, and has fewer and milder side effects. And as we will soon see, St. John's wort has even more to offer in the treatment of depression. It may combine the best of all *three* classes of antidepressant drugs, while also targeting some of the physical causes of depression that prescription antidepressants do not.

❖

Jacqueline's Story: Success over Severe Depression

Jacqueline, a thirty-one-year-old newspaper reporter who specializes in health and science news, knows first-hand the terrible toll depression can take. She grew up watching her mother suffer the ravages of bipolar disease (manic-depression). At the same time, Jacqueline's father was also fighting a losing battle with chronic clinical depression, and he was on and off prescription antidepressants and in and out of psychotherapy for years. Since depression had decimated both sides of Jacqueline's family, she figured it was just a matter of time before it also took hold of her and her older brother.

"Sure enough," Jacqueline says, "my brother began having problems with depression right after he started college. At first his symptoms were mild—trouble sleeping, a vague unhappiness, anxiety. But then the symptoms escalated. He lost interest in his studies, dropped out of school, experienced feelings of hopelessness, talked about ending it all. He tried therapy first, but it wasn't enough. Then he experimented with several different kinds of antidepressants. But most of the drugs he took seemed to give him only a little relief from his symptoms. And the ones that did work better left him with terrible side effects. Eventually he settled on a drug that provided some relief, but the tradeoff in side effects and quality of life was enormous. Plus, he never seemed quite himself again."

Jacqueline got through her teens and early twenties without experiencing any bouts with depression herself. She began to wonder if the disease had "skipped" her. Then, in her late twenties, a move across country and a failed marriage seemed to trigger the first symptoms.

"In the beginning it just felt like free-floating anxiety. All of a sudden I was fearful about things that hadn't bothered me before, and I began to have trouble sleeping at night and getting through the next day. At first I didn't think much about it. I had just made a lot of changes in my life, and I figured a little anxiety was normal."

But Jacqueline's symptoms, like her brother's, soon escalated. "What started as anxiety," she says, "became straight-out fear and a terrible sense that I was losing control of my life. I never slept through the night, had little energy during the day, and, worse, the work that I loved was beginning to suffer. It took me longer and longer to finish an assignment, and I rarely got any enjoyment or satisfaction out of what I did. I seemed to become overly sensitive, especially in work situations, and took even the smallest slights and criticisms way too personally. I also started getting sick all the time and had several bouts with pneumonia, eventually developing chronic bronchitis. Then I began thinking about suicide. At first it was just a fleeting thought, as if I were considering it as a 'last-resort' option. But as my symptoms got worse, and life got darker, and I felt less and less healthy, I began to think about suicide every day."

Jacqueline knew she was suffering from clinical depression, and she knew where that depression could lead. But because of her experiences watching her family deal with depression, largely unsuccessfully, Jacqueline also had very strong feelings about treatment.

"I knew up front that I didn't want to take Prozac or any other prescription antidepressant. I know that's a controversial decision, but it was my personal decision, based on what I saw happen with family members. I had seen just too much of the bad side of prescription antidepressants. I also didn't have a lot of faith in psychotherapy. Again, that's a personal choice. I'm a very private person, and the thought of sitting down with a stranger to talk about these things turned me off."

As an investigative science journalist, Jacqueline had access to the latest research news and medical information about drugs and depression, and she had a deft facility for sifting through medical data and separating fact from fiction. The year before her symptoms became problematic, Jacqueline had come across several German medical journal articles about St. John's wort and depression.

"I went back and reread the German studies, and I was really impressed. Here was a natural drug that had been used successfully in Europe for many years to treat depression, and it had very few, if any, side effects."

In the fall of 1995 Jacqueline began taking St. John's wort daily for her depression. She takes two 325-mg tablets, standarized to 0.3 percent hypericin, one in the morning and one in the early evening.

"It kicked in in two weeks," Jacqueline says. "I felt an enormous difference. I stopped thinking about death, and I stopped taking things so personally. I also had had a lot of sleep disturbances and insomnia, and I don't have either problem anymore. Plus, I have much more physical energy. Most important, I could finally step away from work and see it just as work. Before, work had defined me and controlled me. Now it doesn't. And I haven't had any bad side effects at all. Just one good one: I'm never sick anymore, and my chronic bronchitis has disappeared! In fact, the only problem I have with taking St. John's wort is that sometimes it's hard to get; my local health food store runs out of it very quickly."

We include Jacqueline's story—an incredible success story—even though she breaks most of the rules about taking St. John's wort for depression. For one, St. John's wort is recommended only for mild to moderate depressions. Depressions involving recurrent thoughts of suicide are considered severe, and there has been very little research done on the use of St. John's wort for severe depression. Two, for treating depression, St. John's wort is usually taken under the supervision of a medical practitioner or in tandem with some form of psychotherapy. Jacqueline takes St. John's wort on her own and doesn't see a therapist. Finally, Jacqueline is actually taking slightly less than the recommended total daily dose of St. John's wort, which is 900 mg a day. But this regimen has worked remarkably well for her.

❖

As we mentioned in Chapter 1, St. John's wort has been used medically in traditional Western herbal medicine for almost two thousand years. One of its primary uses for centuries has been as a **nervine**. In herbal medicine, the nervines are plant herbs that nourish and strengthen the nervous system and are used to treat sadness, stress, tension, insomnia, and anxiety, all of which are known symptoms of depression. The nervines also act as "tonics" in the body. That is, they not only treat specific conditions—anxiety, for example—but they simultaneously strengthen ("tone") the body overall by nurturing and supporting the immune system.

While the use of St. John's wort for all its applications fell out of favor for a time in English-speaking countries in the first half of the twentieth century, it was frequently prescribed for its nervine properties in non-English-speaking countries, most notably Germany. There, by the 1980s, it became the most widely used medication for mild-to-moderate depression (prescribed by both conventional *and* alternative practitioners), outselling Prozac, for example, by nearly 50 percent.

With more than 20 million German people taking over 60 million doses of St. John's wort daily, Germany led the way in pioneering research on the herb's effectiveness compared to standard antidepressants, its safety and side effects during use, and the possible biochemical mechanisms by which it worked. The conclusions indicated that compared to conventional antidepressants, St. John's wort was equally effective in treating mild-to-moderate depression, remarkably safe, and significantly less costly. In other parts of the world, researchers, medical practitioners, and people living with depression (not to mention pharmaceutical manufacturers) began to take notice.

During the last twenty years, a wealth of research has been conducted investigating the antidepressant effects of hypericum (St. John's wort) and many of its constituents both *in vitro* and in numerous animal studies and patient trials. To date, hypericum's effectiveness has been studied in more than 5,000 patients in more than twenty-five clinical trials, half of which were double-blind studies. That is, the patients and researchers both did not know which medication was being taken by either study group— hypericum or a conventional antidepressant. The results of all these studies indicate that hypericum is an effective antidepressant for mild-to-moderate depression and is well tolerated by patients.

Based on these initial results, the National Institutes of Health and their Office of Alternative Medicine will soon conduct a multimillion-dollar study of hypericum's antidepressant action in multiple clinical trials throughout the United States. In the meantime, new research findings on hypericum's therapeutic properties are published every few months. We have already highlighted some of those findings in Chapter 2. The balance of this chapter focuses exclusively on the use of hypericum to treat depression.

HOW HYPERICUM TREATS DEPRESSION

While recent research categorically shows that hypericum is a very effective antidepressant, what still isn't clear is just *how* it treats depression. But researchers are getting closer to that answer every day.

The scientific approach to deciphering how hypericum works has typically been a conventional one. Researchers have isolated and tested single chemical constituents of hypericum for their specific therapeutic properties, hoping to find the one or two chemical agents uniquely responsible for its antidepressant actions. We detailed this conventional approach to studying plants in Chapter 2 and pointed out why it's not the best approach to understanding how plant herbs work. Practitioners of traditional herbal medicine believe the therapeutic properties of most plants are dependent on the synergistic interaction of *all* the chemical constituents in the plant.

The most recent research into hypericum's antidepressant properties tends to confirm the traditionalists' point of view. Numerous biochemical studies of the plant's constituents have yielded increasingly diverse information about all of hypericum's therapeutic properties, but particularly about its antidepressant actions. What's particularly interesting about those actions—and unique to hypericum—is that it seems to treat depression on two fronts. It targets biochemical imbalances in the brain just as standard antidepressants do. But hypericum also treats the physical symptoms of depression by boosting the body's immune system. Let's take a brief look at both those actions.

Treating the Brain: The MAOI vs. SSRI Controversy

In early studies of hypericum that occurred in the 1970s, scientists focused on two of the plant's primary chemical constituents, hypericin and pseudohypericin, with hypericin being studied the most frequently. Researchers isolated these constituents from other chemical compounds in the plant and studied them singly, either in natural form or in synthetic variations.

Hypericum as an MAOI. The results of these preliminary studies, which used high doses of the chemical constituents, indicated that both hypericin and pseudohypericin were MAOIs—that is, agents that raised serotonin levels by inhibiting the action of the enzyme monoamine oxidase (which breaks down serotonin). The hypericum plant (along with its primary constituents) was therefore initially labeled an MAOI, similar to Nardil and Parnate. This was mostly good news. The MAOIs are excellent antidepressants, and hypericum has far fewer side effects than prescription MAOIs.

Unfortunately, as noted earlier in this chapter, the MAOIs are also associated with additional and potentially fatal side effects when combined with certain foods and other drugs. Hypericum, as a MAOI-like plant herb, inherited the same negative associations with potentially serious side effects.

Subsequent research pointed out, however, that the earlier research had been erroneous, largely because it used such high doses of hypericin isolated from other constituents in the plant. Nevertheless, much of the hypericum literature, including several books, warns people to avoid the same substances that individuals taking prescription MAOIs do. It's important to note here that there is no evidence, scientific or anecdotal, to support this warning when hypericum is taken at normal doses of 900 mg daily. The MAO-inhibiting effect in hypericum is very mild and just one component of the plant's antidepressant action. Indeed, other constituents in the plant—among them, pseudohypericin, quercitrin, and the xanthones—subsequently exhibited stronger MAO-inhibiting effects than hypericin did, and also at mild levels. They demonstrated other antidepressant properties as well.

Hypericum as an SSRI. In fact, a second wave of research studies in the late 1980s and early to mid-1990s strongly indicated that the antidepressant action of hypericum, in its fully extracted form (with all its plant constituents), was most like Prozac and the other SSRIs, but with milder side effects. This was even better news than the first round of information, because the SSRIs are the best tolerated of the antidepressant drugs. Like Prozac and the other SSRIs, hypericum helps to prevent the reuptake (absorption) of serotonin by brain cells and to keep levels of serotonin high. Hypericum's flavonoids, specifically amentoflavone, the xanthones, and GABA-binding receptors, were all believed to be partly responsible for hypericum's serotonin effect.

Hypericum as an SNDRI? Then a third wave of research studies, some just completed in late 1997, produced even more startling information about hypericum's antidepressant properties. Not only did whole hypericum extracts inhibit serotonin reuptake, they also appeared to directly affect the levels of norepinephrine and dopamine in the brain. These powerful neurotransmitters are crucial to a healthy central nervous system. Now hypericum was looking more like the classic tricyclic antidepressants (TCAs). In fact, in at least one study of more than 200 patients, it outperformed and proved safer than imipramine, the "gold standard" of all antidepressants.

If these latest research results are validated by other studies, hypericum may become the only commercially available antidepressant that acts as a serotonin-norepinephrine-dopamine reuptake inhibitor (SNDRI) and one of the few, if any, therapeutic agents that specifically treats dopamine deficiencies.

Treating the Body: Hypericum as an Immune-Modulator

Russian and German research has confirmed that hypericum is a significant immune-modulator: It both stimulates the immune system when infection and inflammation are present, and suppresses an overstimulated immune system that has been stretched to its maximum capacity by physical and emotional stress. (This is one of the primary reasons why hypericum is also an excellent antiviral and antibacterial agent.)

As is increasingly evident from studies of stress-induced illness, there is a significant link between emotional well-being and physical well-being. As it turns out, the immune system is just as seriously taxed by depression as it is by viral or bacterial infections that threaten the body. In depression, unfortunately, the communication between the brain and the body is often a question of mixed signals that do neither the brain nor the body any good.

The biochemical imbalances in the brain that typify major depression trigger neurotransmitters there to send a message to the immune system that something is wrong throughout the organism. The immune system responds by producing interleukins, the chemical messengers of the immune system that go into alert mode whenever infection threatens healthy cells.

But in depression, the interleukins are really responding to distress signals from the brain, not from the body, and when they cannot find a physical infection to mediate, they send a message back to the immune system center that they need more help. Interleukin production goes into overload, and the body is flooded with confused and misdirected chemical messengers who have nowhere to go and nothing to do but sit there. The integrity of the immune system is compromised and the system effectively shuts down. The body, in turn, is now ripe for opportunistic infections. That is one of the primary reasons why people with major depression are besieged by chronic infections and nonspecific aches and pains.

Hypericum, as a powerful immune-modulator, both decreases the excessive quantities of interleukins throughout the body and strengthens and supports the beleaguered immune system. As interleukin production decreases and the immune system as a whole is restored to balance, many of the physical symptoms associated with a person's depression are relieved. In fact, with hypericum, the physical symptoms of depression are often the first to go. This is another aspect of the plant's antidepressant action that is, like its SNDRI-effect, totally unique to hypericum.

Much of this new research is extraordinary news indeed for the millions of people who live with depression, even when further studies are definitely called for.

What is important to repeat here is that based on all these research studies, there is absolutely no doubt about hypericum's effectiveness in treating mild-to-moderate depression for a significant number of people. And it treats such depressions safely, inexpensively, and with far fewer and milder side effects than prescription antidepressants. So let's move on to the who, what, when, and how of treating depression with hypericum.

USING HYPERICUM TO TREAT *YOUR* DEPRESSION

Depression is a serious disease, and hypericum is potent medicine. These two facts cannot be repeated often enough.

Too much of recent mainstream literature about St. John's wort has a "jump on the bandwagon" mentality. Some writers and alternative medicine advocates seem to suggest that just because hypericum is a natural herb with mild side effects it can be used by anyone who is experiencing some depressive symptoms. This simply isn't true.

In the most scientifically rigorous of the clinical trials involving patients, hypericum was effective in 75 percent of cases at the most. And these were patients who had been thoroughly evaluated by medical doctors beforehand, who had received a clinical diagnosis of major depression, and who were closely monitored throughout the trials. Depression is difficult to treat, and finding the optimal antidepressant for a person's unique set of symptoms is often the most difficult part of that treatment. Like the synthetic antidepressants, hypericum is not always effective in treating some mild-to-moderate depressions.

With those warnings, please bear the following in mind . . .

- If You Are Already Taking a Prescription Antidepressant
  —Don't stop taking it! If you are interested in using hypericum as an alternative antidepressant, talk to your medical practitioner first. All the pro-and-con scientific evidence about mixing hypericum with other antidepressants isn't in yet. Some research implies that hypericum can be used as adjunctive (supportive) therapy with a serotonin reuptake inhibitor, such as Prozac, but we do not recommend it. Other research strongly suggests that it is best to gradually withdraw from a prescription antidepressant before beginning a treatment regimen with hypericum. Again, working with a qualified medical practitioner—conventional or alternative—is the best and safest course of action when switching from a conventional drug to hypericum.

- If You Suspect You Have a Depressive Disorder
  —Don't self-medicate with hypericum! Review the guidelines for major depression (listed earlier in this chapter), then talk to a qualified medical practitioner to get a thorough evaluation of your symptoms. Remember, hypericum has been tested only in patients with mild-to-moderate depressions. Also, many milder forms of depression don't require an antidepressant at all; psychotherapy alone can pro-

duce wonderful results in some cases. The bottom line here is that hypericum is medicine, and you shouldn't take medicine you don't need.

- If You Have Mild-to-Moderate Depression and You Are Working with a Qualified Medical Practitioner
  —*Do* try hypericum after reviewing all your treatment options and after discussing with your practitioner other medications you may be taking or other medical conditions you may have, such as high blood pressure. Also review our descriptions of the possible side effects of hypericum in Chapter 2 and our guidelines for buying and using research-grade hypericum in Chapter 3. The most up-to-date research on hypericum and depression recommends the following as optimal daily doses for treating mild-to-moderate depression:

Tablet or Capsule Forms: 300 mg of hypericum extract standardized to 0.3 percent hypericin, 3 times a day with meals, for a total of 900 mg daily.

Liquid Extract Form: 1/4 teaspoon (approximately 20 drops) of hypericum extract standardized to 0.3 percent hypericin, 3 times a day in distilled water, with meals, for a total of 3/4 teaspoon daily.

Like the other antidepressants, hypericum is a slow-acting therapeutic agent. You should wait at least four to six weeks for its full antidepressant effects to be felt. However, you may notice some physical effects sooner than that.

- Improved sleep patterns may occur as early as seven days after beginning treatment. Furthermore, hypericum does not interfere with normal dream patterns, as do prescription antidepressants, nor does it produce the intense and vivid dreams associated with prescription medications.

- Eating disorders, including both poor appetite and overeating, may improve as early as two weeks after beginning treatment.

- Fatigue, exhaustion, and low energy levels may also improve as early as two weeks after beginning treatment.

- The "blues" or depressed mood may improve as early as three weeks after beginning treatment.

- A general sense of well-being may also occur as early as three weeks after beginning treatment.

After you have been on hypericum for a while, you will probably also notice that you feel physically stronger and healthier. And, in fact, you may well be. Hypericum's potent immune-modulating properties, as well as its antiviral and antibacterial action, may make you more resistant to run-of-the-mill colds and viruses and help you recover quickly when they do occur. This is another "bonus" of hypericum treatment that other antidepressants don't offer.

Length of Treatment: Current research strongly suggests that hypericum be taken for no more than a year. This recommended duration of treatment is actually standard for all the antidepressants.

What to Do if Side Effects Occur: If bothersome side effects occur while you are taking hypericum, you do not have to taper off the herb, as with some other antidepressants. It can be stopped immediately. If you are going to try another antidepressant, however, you and your practitioner should wait the recommended two to four weeks before beginning a new treatment regimen, particularly if you are planning to use one of the serotonin-based drugs.

USING HYPERICUM TO TREAT SEASONAL AFFECTIVE DISORDER

Seasonal affective disorder (SAD)—also known as "major depression with seasonal pattern," "seasonal depression," or simply the "winter blues"—is a subtype of major depression that generally occurs in the late fall or winter and completely disappears in the spring. It seems to be related to decreasing sunlight as the winter days grow shorter.

The symptoms of SAD are the same as those for mild-to-moderate depression, and include mood swings, depressed mood, sadness, fatigue, general physical debilitation, sleep disorders (especially oversleeping), eating disorders (especially overeating and craving sweets and starches), weight gain, and listlessness.

Conventional Treatments of SAD

Conventional treatments of SAD include a number of the same antidepressant medicines used in treating mild-to-moderate depression, phototherapy, or a combination of medication and phototherapy.

Phototherapy, also called light therapy, has become the preferred treatment option. It is a fairly new therapeutic approach that was devised because SAD occurs primarily during the winter months and is believed to be related to diminishing sunlight. Phototherapy treatment involves exposing people with SAD to a very bright and broad-spectrum artificial light that contains all the wavelengths of sunlight. The light is dispersed by means of a special box or by a visor that attaches to the individual's head.

Phototherapy treatment is usually monitored by a specialist in that field, although portable home devices are also available. Treatment sessions are generally administered on a daily basis for thirty minutes to two hours per session, depending on the severity of symptoms. Phototherapy on its own is quite effective for some people, though other individuals may need a combination of antidepressants and light therapy to relieve their symptoms fully.

One drawback of phototherapy is that it can be quite time-consuming and intrusive. Another concern is that its long-term side effects are not known since it is a relatively new treatment form, and there is some concern that permanent eye damage may be a problem. Short-term side effects of phototherapy may include headache, irritability, strained eyes, and sleep disturbances.

Treating SAD with Hypericum

Hypericum's effectiveness in treating SAD was documented in a 1994 single-blind study conducted in Germany, where hypericum has long been used to treat the symptoms of seasonal affective disorder.

Two groups of outpatients who had been diagnosed with SAD were each prescribed hypericum (300 mg, 3 times a day). One group also received broad-spectrum phototherapy for two hours each day. The other group received a nontherapeutic "dim" light treatment that mimicked phototherapy.

At the end of four weeks, both groups of patients showed a significant improvement in their depressive symptoms (based on the Hamilton Depression Rating Scale) and experienced minimal side effects. Furthermore, there was no significant difference in improvement rates between the two groups. In other words, the patients who received only hypericum improved just as much as those patients who received hypericum *and* phototherapy!

Based on the results of this specific study, as well as the larger body of research on hypericum and major depression, you may want to try using hypericum alone for your SAD symptoms—under a practitioner's care, of course. We recommend that the following daily doses be taken for a six-month period, from September through March.

Tablet or Capsule Forms: 300 mg of hypericum extract standardized to 0.3 percent hypericin, 3 times a day with meals, for a total of 900 mg daily.

Liquid Extract Form: 1/4 teaspoon (approximately 20 drops) of hypericum extract standardized to 0.3 percent hypericin, 3 times a day in distilled water, with meals, for a total of 3/4 teaspoon daily.

Since the full effects of hypericum may not be felt for four to six weeks, we recommend you start taking it in early September. That way, by the time the days begin to shorten significantly, you will be receiving the full therapeutic effects of the herb.

ST. JOHN'S WORT CALMING TEA
❖

This is a soothing tea for body and soul during stressful times or when you are feeling especially anxious. Use dried herb for the ingredients.

  2 teaspoons St. John's wort
  1 teaspoon rosehips
  1 teaspoon balm
  1 teaspoon valerian
  4–5 cups pure spring water, boiled

Place all the dried herb ingredients in a large glass or enameled teapot that you have prewarmed with hot water. (Discard the hot water before adding herbs.) Pour boiling spring water over the herbs, cover the pot, and allow the tea to steep for 15 minutes. Strain into a cup or mug and season to taste with honey.

Drink 3 to 4 cups of this tea throughout the day, evenly spaced between meals. You may leave the pot out on your kitchen counter and drink the tea at room temperature. If you prefer your tea hot, gently warm (not boil) the tea in a glass or enameled pot on top of the stove, or add 1–2 teaspoons boiling water to a cup of lukewarm tea. Never microwave herbal tea. Discard any leftover teas and grounds at the end of the day.

ST. JOHN'S WORT RESTORATIVE TEA
❖

This tea is a true tonic. It has both a balancing effect on
the emotions and an energizing effect on the body and
brain. It's especially good for those days when you are
feeling physically low and mentally fuzzy but still need
to get things done! Use dried herb for the ingredients.

>   2 teaspoons St. John's wort
>   1 teaspoon lavender
>   1 teaspoon peppermint
>   1 teaspoon rosemary
>   4–5 cups pure spring water, boiled

Place all the dried herb ingredients in a large glass or
enameled teapot that you have prewarmed with hot water. (Discard the hot water before adding herbs.) Pour
boiling spring water over the herbs, cover the pot, and
allow the tea to steep for 15 minutes. Strain into a cup
or mug and season to taste with honey.

Drink 3 to 4 cups of this tea throughout the day, evenly
spread between meals. You may leave the pot out on
your kitchen counter and drink the tea at room temperature. If you prefer your tea hot, gently warm (not
boil) the tea in a glass or enameled pot on top of the
stove, or add 1–2 teaspoons boiling water to a cup of
lukewarm tea. Never microwave herbal tea. Discard
any leftover teas and grounds at the end of the day.

Depression is a daunting and insidious disease—for those who live with it, who live around it, and who treat it. Not only is it difficult to diagnose and treat, it may also go unrecognized for years on end, effectively placing a stranglehold on millions of human lives during their most formative and productive years.

But this is one serious medical condition that is highly treatable and often curable. There are many treatment options available to those who live with depression, not the least of which, now, is hypericum. The appearance of St. John's wort on the therapeutic landscape, as an effective, natural, safe, and inexpensive antidepressant, may be the most heartening medical development to occur in the field of depression for years.

Remember, too, that depression is a quintessentially body-mind-spirit disease, with physical, mental, and emotional components. Alternative medicine, therefore, with its emphasis on holistic treatment and total health, has much to offer in the support of depression, besides the benefits of hypericum.

For one, many other herbs combine well with hypericum in teas and tonics, which can provide additional short-term support during treatment for depression. Some herbs sharing hypericum's calming properties are valerian *(Valeriana officinalis)*, lobelia *(Lobelia inflata)*, hops *(Humulus lupulus)*, rosehips *(Rosa canina)*, and balm *(Melissa officinalis)*. Herbs that share hypericum's immune-strengthening and energy-enhancing actions are echinacea *(Echinacea augustifolia)*, ginseng *(Panax schinseng)*, ginger *(Zingiber officinale)*, and cinnamon *(Cinnamomum zeylanicum)*. Check your local health food stores for teas and tonics containing these herbs, or try one of the recipes we share in this chapter.

Good nutrition, nutritional supplements, gentle body-mind exercises (such as t'ai chi), chiropractic manipulation, massage, and meditation techniques all add immeasurably to physical and emotional well-being. Many of the reference books listed in the back of the book, particularly those under Chapter 1, provide wonderful instruction in using the therapeutic tools of alternative medicine to help treat depression.

CHAPTER 6

❖

Treating PMS, Menstrual Problems, and Menopausal Symptoms with St. John's Wort

Until quite recently, women carried the plant during wartime, in the hope that it would prevent their violation.
— FROM THE CHAPTER ON
"ST. JOHN'S WORT" IN *HERBALISM* BY FRANK J. LIPP

It may feel like war, even violation—the inevitable, sometimes subtle, often seismic ebb and flow of hormones that characterize premenstrual syndrome (PMS), menstruation, and menopause. These changes may be natural, even empowering for some, but they are life-disrupting for many.

The one to two weeks of wide-ranging physical, emotional, and mental discomfort that precede menstruation may affect work and family life, friendships, critical thinking, and sleep patterns. The cramps, nausea, and diarrhea that accompany many menstrual periods are physically and emotionally debilitating. The hot flashes, rapid heartbeat, numb extremities, pounding headaches, and pronounced anxiety and fatigue that frequently signal menopause may lay many a woman low just as she is hitting her stride professionally and socially.

Women ride the waves of profound hormonal sea changes for most of their lives. From as young as 9 to as old as 60, they live the truth that health and well-being are equal parts body and soul.

• • •

For centuries hypericum has been prized as a "woman's tonic," both for its effectiveness in treating specific menstrual and menopausal symptoms and for its unique ability to strengthen ("tone") the entire reproductive system. In ancient times, in fact, hypericum's effectiveness as a woman's tonic was almost as well known as its esteemed wound-healing and infection-fighting properties. It is one of a special group of plants—traditionally known as emmenagogues and uterine tonics—that have a long history of successful use in treating women's disorders.

A Mini-Primer on Herbs As Female Tonics

In traditional herbal medicine, the emmenagogues are plant herbs that regulate menstruation by promoting and increasing menstrual flow through stimulation of the uterus. Many people erroneously think of the emmenagogues as synonymous with abortifacients, plants and drugs that induce abortion. Some of the stronger emmenagogues—pennyroyal *(Mentha pulegium)*, juniper *(Juniperus communis)*, goldenseal *(Hydrastis canadensis)*, and barberry *(Berberis vulgaris)*, among others—have been used in large doses for that purpose.

Hypericum is a mild emmenagogue that helps regulate menstruation, but it is not an abortifacient. However, any plant herb that may stimulate uterine contractions should, of course, be avoided during pregnancy or if you are trying to conceive. (See Chapter 3 for more specific information on hypericum's side effects.)

Besides being an emmenagogue, hypericum is also, and perhaps most importantly, a uterine tonic. The uterine tonics are plant herbs that tone, nurture, and strengthen the organs and tissues of the reproductive system and support optimal gynecologic health. Some of the uterine tonics are stimulating in overall effect and are used to promote proper ovarian function and regulate menstruation; rue *(Ruta graveolens)* and blue cohosh *(Caulophyllum thalictroides)* are good examples of this type of uterine tonic. Other plants have a relaxing effect on the uterus and are used to treat cramps and muscle spasms and to prevent miscarriage; the aptly named cramp bark *(Virburnum opulus)* is one example of such a plant. Still other plant herbs appear to have a direct hormonal influence on the reproductive system and have been used to treat menopausal symptoms and infertility; examples are wild yam *(Dioscorea villosa)* and false unicorn root *(Chamaelirion luteum)*. A final group of plant herbs nourish and support the reproductive system by promoting healthy biochemical functioning on a cellular level; chaste tree *(Vitex agnus-castus)* is an excellent example of an all-around uterine tonic.

Hypericum: A Multipurpose Female Tonic

Hypericum shares many of the therapeutic properties of *all* the uterine tonics. It helps normalize and promote menstruation and relieves pain and spasms. It also provides overall support to organs and tissues by regulating some of the biochemical actions of the reproductive system, notably the production of excess prostaglandins that cause many of the symptoms of PMS, as well as painful cramps and heavy bleeding during menstruation. Hypericum may even have a mild hormonal effect. Studies of its chemical constituents have identified at least one estrogenic agent, beta-sitosterol, a basic building block used in the synthesis of several hormones, including estrogen, which also is found in wild yams and soybeans.

Hypericum has several other healing properties that contribute significantly to its role as a female tonic. It has

superb anti-inflammatory action, is an excellent yet mild
diuretic *and* antidiarrheal, and has a proven track record
in treating anxiety, fatigue, sleep disturbances, and depressed moods.

Most current research on hypericum has focused on
its antidepressant, antiviral, antibacterial, and anticancer
properties, and so there is little clinical data on its use in
treating PMS or menstrual and menopausal symptoms.
Still, based on hypericum's other clinically validated therapeutic actions, as well as its long traditional use as a female
tonic and substantial anecdotal information, we can make
some reasonable suppositions about its potential benefits
for treating some of the common symptoms and discomfort
associated with PMS, menstruation, and menopause.

First we define each condition, describe its basic symptoms, and look at conventional treatments for it. Then we
discuss hypericum's potential effectiveness in treating the
condition and recommend how and when to use it.

❖

Marjorie's Story:
PMS Relief—A Positive Side Effect

Marjorie, a thirty-two-year-old computer analyst who
has experienced chronic moderate depression for ten
years with only minimal relief of her symptoms, started
taking St. John's wort in combination with the prescription antidepressant, Zoloft, about a year and a half ago.
While she was thrilled to find that the combination
treatment almost completely relieved her depression,
Marjorie was equally happy to discover that the addition of St. John's wort to her treatment regimen deliv-
ered an unexpected bonus.

"For years I've suffered from severe PMS, together

with irregular and painful menstrual periods. I had terrible mood swings, headaches, and insomnia with the PMS, and very heavy bleeding and cramping with my periods. I even had a couple of D&Cs, but they had little effect on my symptoms. However, since I've been on the St. John's wort, for the first time in my life I've had almost no PMS symptoms and regular periods as well! I rarely have mood swings or headaches before my periods, and besides being regular, I don't have heavy bleeding or painful cramping anymore. I'm convinced this is the result of the St. John's wort, since it's the only new thing I've added to my treatment in years. And I intend to keep taking it."

❖

TREATING PMS WITH HYPERICUM

What Is PMS?

PMS is a constellation of symptoms that classically begin anywhere from one to two weeks before the start of the menstrual period and then gradually stop with the onset of menstruation. PMS affects about 50 percent of all women between the ages of 25 and 40, with as many as nine out of ten women experiencing some mild symptoms from time to time and other women experiencing chronic and debilitating symptoms on a regular basis.

What Are the Symptoms of PMS?

The symptoms of PMS are various and affect many parts of the body at the same time, including the reproductive, gastrointestinal, and central nervous system. PMS symptoms may include the following:

- Fluid retention (bloating), constipation, and/or diarrhea
- Swollen (puffy) ankles or hands
- Swollen and painful breasts
- Headaches
- Anxiety, nervousness, sadness
- Irritability and anger
- Light-headedness or dizziness (occasionally fainting)
- Extreme fatigue
- Sleep disturbances (oversleeping or insomnia)
- Skin disturbances (extremely dry skin and/or acne)
- Scanty urination
- Changes in sexual drive

Some women also report being more susceptible to viral infections, such as colds and flus, during this time, and having more minor accidents (due to clumsiness and fatigue). Women are also significantly more susceptible to the effects of alcohol during the premenstrual period.

What Are the Causes of PMS?

There is no one cause of PMS. Instead, several factors seem to be involved. These include extreme changes in levels of the hormones estrogen and progesterone, which affect the reproductive, digestive, cardiovascular, and central nervous systems, as well as the skin and bones.

During the premenstrual period there is also increased production of prostaglandins, highly active biochemical substances released from organ and tissue cells when there is injury or stimulation (such as changes in hormone levels). The prostaglandins, carried through the blood stream, have wide-ranging effects in the body, including stimulating the intestines and other smooth muscles, changing heart rate and blood pressure, and causing the uterus to contract. They also "antagonize" (inhibit) the action of several key neurotransmitters in the brain that affect mood, including epinephrine and norepinephrine.

In addition to these major biochemical changes in the body during the two weeks leading up to menstruation, other key players contribute to the symptoms of PMS: stress, diet, and lifestyle.

Conventional Treatments of PMS

There is no one mode of treatment—or any one drug— that is completely effective in relieving PMS. In general, various medications, together with diet and lifestyle counseling, are recommended.

Among the prescription medications that are sometimes prescribed to alleviate the symptoms of PMS are tranquilizers and antianxiety drugs, oral contraceptives, and diuretics. Danocrine (danazol), a prescription drug designed specifically to treat endometriosis (the painful overgrowth of the uterine lining), is sometimes prescribed for PMS, but it can also produce disturbing side effects, such as facial hair and a deepening voice.

Women with PMS also are frequently advised by their medical practitioners to avoid stress or precipitators of stress, to limit their salt and caffeine intake, to avoid alcohol, to exercise moderately, and to seek counseling or group support. Diet and nutritional counseling include recommendations to avoid fats and eat high-complex carbohydrates.

Vitamin supplementation may also be helpful, including

vitamins A and D for skin problems, vitamins C and E for physical and emotional stress, and vitamin B6 to increase energy and to help relieve bloating, moodiness, and sugar cravings. Supplemental calcium and selenium (for muscle cramps and pain) and magnesium (for mood swings) may also be recommended.

Using Hypericum to Treat PMS

Hypericum appears to have much to offer in treating many of the symptoms of PMS. In particular, hypericum's diuretic, astringent, analgesic, anti-inflammatory, sedating, immune-modulating, and prostaglandin-inhibiting actions may all combine to provide comprehensive PMS relief. Let's look at how each of these actions can relieve the symptoms of PMS.

- **Diuretic and Astringent Action.** Hypericum's diuretic action promotes urination and may help eliminate the abdominal bloating and swollen breasts, ankles, and hands of PMS. Its astringent action may help with PMS-related diarrhea.

- **Analgesic Action.** Hypericum is a proven pain reliever and has been used in the treatment of chronic tension headaches and neuralgia (nerve pain). Thus it may help relieve the pounding headaches and lower back pain that frequently accompany PMS.

- **Anti-inflammatory Action.** Hypericum has clinically documented anti-inflammatory action that also may help relieve headaches and lower back pain as well as painful and swollen breasts, ankles, and hands.

- **Sedating Action.** There is substantial clinical evidence confirming hypericum's sedating, antianxiety, antidepressant, and sleep-promoting actions, all of which can go far in relieving the anxiety, irritability, moodiness, and sleep disturbances commonly associated with PMS.

- **Immune-Modulating Action.** As discussed in the chapter on depression, hypericum appears to be a significant immune-system modulator. It both stimulates the immune system in the presence of infection and inflammation, and suppresses an overactive immune system that is taxed by physical and emotional stressors. The profound biochemical changes that characterize PMS, menstruation, and menopause are themselves significant stressors in the body. Hypericum's immune-stimulating action can strengthen the body's defenses against the opportunistic infections that women are more prone to during PMS. Its immune-suppressing action may relieve inflammation-related pain and discomfort, as well as moodiness and fatigue.

- **Prostaglandin-Inhibiting Action.** As mentioned earlier in the chapter, prostaglandin production increases dramatically during the premenstrual period, stimulated in part by changes in hormone levels. Prostaglandin activity affects how one feels physically and mentally. Overproduction of prostaglandins is associated with uncomfortable changes in mood, heart rate, blood pressure, and muscle contraction. Hypericum's prostaglandin-inhibiting action—also a key factor in the plant's antidepressant properties—may help relieve some of the moodiness and physical discomfort

associated with PMS by decreasing or stabilizing
prostaglandin production.

Hypericum appears to have great therapeutic potential for
treating many of the symptoms of PMS. If you would
like to try hypericum for your own PMS symptoms, we
strongly advise you to consult with a qualified medical
practitioner and discuss with him or her any preexisting
medical conditions you may have or any alternative or
conventional medications you are already taking.

You should also review the side effects and contraindications for hypericum listed in Chapter 3. Finally, avoid taking hypericum (or any other nonprescribed plant or
synthetic medication) at all, if you are trying to become
pregnant. If you and your practitioner feel comfortable
with your taking hypericum, our recommendations for
how and when to use it are below.

How and When to Use Hypericum for PMS

Try adding hypericum to your daily self-care regimen
about two weeks after the first day of your last menstrual
period. For tablet or capsule form, take 300 mg of hypericum extract 3 times a day with meals, for a total of
900 mg daily. For liquid form, take 1/4 teaspoon (approximately 20 drops) of hypericum extract 3 times a day in a
glass of distilled water, with meals, for a total of 3/4 of a
teaspoon daily. Both tablet and liquid forms of hypericum
should be marked on the label as standarized to 0.3 percent hypericin.

Continue taking hypericum until the start of your menstrual period, then stop taking it when your menstrual
flow begins. (See below for using hypericum during your
menstrual period.) Begin taking hypericum again two

weeks after the last day of your period. You may need to be on this two-weeks-on/two-weeks-off regimen for two to three months before feeling the full effects of hypericum on your PMS symptoms. For this dosage and duration of treatment, hypericum is exceptionally safe and mild-acting. Of course, stop taking hypericum immediately if you experience any significant side effects. And if you continue on this regimen of hypericum treatment, remember always to advise your medical practitioners that you are taking hypericum.

TREATING MENSTRUAL PROBLEMS WITH HYPERICUM

Some Common Menstrual Problems

Four of the most common menstrual problems are:

Dysmenorrhea Severe abdominal pain and cramping at the time of menstruation

Menorrhagia Heavy bleeding during menstruation

Amenorrhea The absence of menstruation

Metrorrhagia Unexpected bleeding between periods

Amenorrhea and metrorrhagia are the less common of the four menstrual problems and are best evaluated by an expert in obstetric and gynecologic care because of the possibility of pregnancy, miscarriage, or potentially serious underlying medical disorders. Menorrhagia, or heavy bleeding during the period, is a common menstrual complaint. Often there is no underlying disorder to explain it, although anemia can be a serious associated illness because of loss of blood. Heavy bleeding may, however, also be a sign of a potentially serious condition and should always be evaluated by a medical practitioner.

In this book, therefore, our focus is solely on hypericum's therapeutic potential for treating dysmenorrhea, the most common menstrual complaint. However, if you regularly experience heavy bleeding during your periods (saturating one sanitary pad or tampon approximately every hour throughout the day), and your medical practitioner has ruled out any underlying cause, you may want to try hypericum for its excellent astringent properties. All the astringent herbs, periwinkle *(Vinca major)*, shepherd's purse *(Capsella bursa-pastoris)*, and lady's mantle *(Alchemilla vulgaris)*, but particularly hypericum, are excellent treatments for stopping excessive blood flow. (They are also effective for diarrhea.) Follow the dosage and duration recommendations we give below for using hypericum to treat dysmenorrhea.

DYSMENORRHEA

Dysmenorrhea is marked by severe abdominal pain and cramping right before and/or during the first day or two of menstruation. There are two types of dysmenorrhea, primary and secondary.

- **Primary dysmenorrhea** is characterized by severe abdominal pain and cramping that occur in the first day or two of the menstrual period. Usually there is a long history of primary dysmenorrhea, often starting with a woman's first periods. It is most prevalent among younger women who have not had a child, and while pregnancy and/or age often resolve dysmenorrhea symptoms, you don't have to wait for either of those eventualities to experience relief.

- **Secondary dysmenorrhea** is characterized by pain and cramping that begin about a week *before* the menstrual period is due and intensify until the period begins. Then they may either stop altogether or worsen with bleeding. Secondary dysmenorrhea occurs years after menstruation begins and is considered a symptom of another underlying disease or condition, including endometriosis, pelvic inflammatory disease, or fibroids, among others.

  Since treatment of secondary dysmenorrhea involves targeting the underlying cause, our treatment recommendations focus on common primary dysmenorrhea where an underlying organic problem has been ruled out.

Any dysmenorrhea that persists over many months, however, despite treatment attempts, should be carefully evaluated by a qualified medical practitioner.

Symptoms of Primary Dysmenorrhea

The symptoms of primary dysmenorrhea may include:

- Severe abdominal cramping and pain at the beginning and/or during menstruation
- Severe cramp-like pain that radiates to the lower back and legs
- Nausea and possible vomiting
- Diarrhea

- Dizziness and occasionally fainting
- Excessive sweating
- General fatigue and debilitation

Causes of Primary Dysmenorrhea

As with PMS, there is no one cause of primary dysmenor-rhea. Biochemical changes in the body, together with stress, diet, and lifestyle factors, all contribute to the symp-toms of primary dysmenorrhea.

On the biochemical front (and as mentioned earlier), prostaglandin production is triggered during this period in part by changes in hormone levels. The prostaglandins are highly active biochemicals that significantly affect smooth muscle contraction, emotional mood, heart rate, and blood pressure. Excessive prostaglandin production is as-sociated with painful muscle contractions and with mood swings. Clinical research has in fact demonstrated that women with primary dysmenorrhea have a significantly higher level of prostaglandins circulating through their blood, and this is considered a primary cause of the severe and painful abdominal muscle cramping that occurs with menstruation.

A family history of dysmenorrhea also appears to be a contributing factor, as do lack of exercise together with physical and emotional stress. Too much caffeine and a generally poor diet can also exacerbate the symptoms of dysmenorrhea.

Conventional Treatments of Primary Dysmenorrhea

Conventional treatments of primary dysmenorrhea focus almost exclusively on relieving the severe pain and muscle contractions. For pain and muscle contractions, the NSAIDs (nonsteroidal anti-inflammatory drugs, such as over-the-counter ibuprofens) are often recommended. The NSAIDs are synthetic prostaglandin-inhibitors.

Dietary counseling is sometimes given, including warnings to avoid caffeine and alcohol, although there are no specific foods that either exacerbate or relieve the symptoms of dysmenorrhea. Nutritional supplementation with calcium, potassium, and magnesium (for muscle pains and muscle contractions), may help ease cramping and pain.

Finally, strenuous and regular exercise, particularly exercise that stretches and tones the pelvic muscles, can be very helpful in reducing abdominal pain and cramping.

Using Hypericum to Treat Primary Dysmenorrhea

Hypericum has a long history of treating the specific discomforts of menstruation. Of particular importance in treating primary dysmenorrhea are hypericum's analgesic, prostaglandin-inhibiting, astringent, anti-inflammatory, and sedating actions.

- **Analgesic Action.** Hypericum has been used effectively to relieve headache pain, nerve pain, and muscle pain. It is also helpful in directly relieving the abdominal and lower back pain that characterize primary dysmenorrhea.

- **Prostaglandin-Inhibiting Action.** As mentioned earlier in the chapter, excessive prostaglandin production, which causes severe pain, muscle contractions, and mood swings, is a major cause of primary dysmenorrhea. Clinical studies have proven that women who experience dysmenorrhea do indeed produce too many prostaglandins. Therefore, hypericum's prostaglandin-inhibiting action may significantly relieve the two primary symptoms of dysmenorrhea, cramping and muscle pain.

- **Astringent Action.** Hypericum's astringent action may help control the diarrhea that often accompanies dysmenorrhea, normalize blood flow and blood clotting, and also help soothe and heal inflamed tissues and muscles.

- **Anti-inflammatory Action.** Hypericum has clinically proven anti-inflammatory properties that contribute significantly to the herb's pain-relieving action. These anti-inflammatory properties also help soothe swollen, damaged, and stressed tissues and muscles.

- **Sedating Action.** The severe pain and cramping that characterize dysmenorrhea are physically and emotionally debilitating and may greatly affect mood, general well-being, and sleep. Hypericum's proven sedating, antianxiety, and sleep-promoting actions promote physical and emotional well-being in women dealing with dysmenorrhea and may calm muscle contractions.

If you would like to try hypericum for the painful cramping of dysmenorrhea, we suggest you first talk with a qualified medical practitioner about any preexisting (or underlying) medical conditions you may have or about any alternative or conventional medications you are already taking that may be contraindicated with hypericum. Also review hypericum's side effects in Chapter 3. If you have done all that, and you feel comfortable taking hypericum, here are our recommendations for how and when to use it.

How and When to Use
Hypericum for Primary Dysmenorrhea

Try adding hypericum to your daily self-care regimen about 7 to 10 days before the scheduled start of your next menstrual period. For tablet or capsule form, take 300 mg of hypericum extract 3 times a day with meals, for a total of 900 mg daily. For liquid form, take 1/4 teaspoon (approximately 20 drops) of hypericum extract 3 times a day in a glass of distilled water, with meals, for a total of 3/4 of a teaspoon daily. Both tablet and liquid forms of hypericum should be marked on the label as standardized to 0.3 percent hypericin.

Continue taking hypericum until the start of your menstrual period, and for the next 1 or 2 days after (or until cramping subsides). Begin taking hypericum again 7 to 10 days before the start of your next menstrual period. You may need to be on this treatment regimen for 2 to 3 months before feeling the full effects of hypericum on your dysmenorrhea. Depending on the severity of your symptoms, you may have to adjust both the dosage of hypericum and the length of time you take it, but don't do this on your own. Instead, we again strongly suggest that you work with a qualified practitioner.

TREATING MENOPAUSAL
SYMPTOMS WITH HYPERICUM

What Is Menopause?

In classic medical terms, menopause is defined as the complete cessation of menstrual periods, which commonly occurs anywhere between the mid-40s and the mid-50s.

In reality, menopause is a conglomerate of symptoms

that occur in stages and may begin, mildly and infrequently, as early as 40, and then continue with increasing intensity and frequency for up to ten years or more until menstruation permanently stops. These symptoms and their stages are variously called perimenopause, premenopause, and menopause, although there is no clearly defined line between the stages and much overlap of symptoms. This can make both the diagnosis and treatment of menopause difficult.

Almost all cultures view menopause as a natural midlife transition for women whose reproductive cycles have dominated their biological lives for thirty to forty years. But it is also a physically and emotionally complex transition that affects not only the reproductive system but every other body system as well, including skin, bones, body tissues, metabolism, emotional well-being, and sexuality. The cardiovascular and central nervous systems are particularly affected as drastically dropping hormone levels frequently cause constriction of the arteries that carry blood and other biochemicals to and from the heart and brain.

The symptoms we describe below have all been associated with the different stages of menopause. Those symptoms that occur infrequently and are only mildly uncomfortable may signal *perimenopause*, particularly if menstrual periods are only somewhat irregular. The same symptoms may increase in frequency and intensity as menstrual periods become more irregular and scant, a time often referred to as *premenopause*. The symptoms may reach maximum frequency and intensity, and often become debilitating, after menstrual periods have ceased for nearly a year—a signal that *menopause* has occurred. Unfortunately, the symptoms may then go on for several years or more after that. Luckily, there is much that conventional and alternative medicine has to offer in the way of treatment.

A full discussion of the physiological components of menopause and the many treatments for it—both alternative and conventional—is beyond the scope of this work. There are numerous books written on menopause alone, and many excellent ones that approach the treatment of menopause from a herbal and holistic perspective. Our focus here is on how hypericum may help treat menopausal symptoms.

We cannot emphasize enough, however, how important it is that you work with a qualified medical practitioner who has expertise in reproductive health if you believe you are experiencing menopausal symptoms. First, you will want to rule out any other medical problems that might be causing your symptoms. Second, the cumulative effect of the many varying symptoms of menopause, together with the changes that they presage, can significantly impact general well-being, family life, social life, and career. More importantly, maintaining optimal physical health and paying special attention to preventive health care is critical around menopause and afterwards.

Estrogen and progesterone, the hormones whose production dramatically decreases with menopause, provide natural protection in menstruating women against three debilitating and potentially fatal conditions—heart disease, stroke, and osteoporosis. Without the protection of estrogen in particular, women are at significantly increased risk for these diseases. Heart disease, in particular, is still notoriously underdiagnosed in women, yet it kills more women each year than any other disease, including breast cancer. For that reason alone, menopause, however natural a transition, should never be taken lightly.

❖

Maria's Story: A Helping Hand During Major Life Changes

Maria, a homemaker whose youngest child had just started college, began taking St. John's wort only a month ago, but already she's singing its praises.

Maria began experiencing some mild depressive symptoms after her fiftieth birthday. Just as her "nest" was finally emptying—giving her and her husband some much-needed and long-anticipated private time together—Maria was hit with a milestone birthday, menopause, and an all-too-quiet house after thirty years of raising four children. Her menopausal symptoms were moderate, and she was able to manage most of them with some changes in diet, nutritional supplements, and a daily walking routine. But for the first time in her busy life, Maria was having trouble sleeping through the night—night after night. Plus she couldn't shake a feeling of free-floating anxiety and dread during the day, and she felt increasingly drained of energy. Then a friend in her monthly reading circle confided that she had been taking a plant herb, St. John's wort, for depression for over a year and had never felt better. Her friend had first heard about the herb from a family member who lived in Europe, where it was widely prescribed, and recently she had seen several magazine articles about it. She told Maria that not only did she sleep like a baby now, but she had more energy and more enthusiasm for life. And she never felt "drugged."

Maria hadn't thought of herself as "technically" depressed, but she saw right away that she had some of the same symptoms her friend had had. A longtime believer in natural health care remedies, Maria was otherwise very healthy, and she decided to give St. John's wort a try. Much to her surprise, she was able to find it easily in the vitamin section of her local drugstore.

"I've been taking three 300-mg capsules three times a day for the last four weeks. And just last week I began to feel some real changes. First of all, I slept through the night for the first time in months—and I mean a really good sleep! And that's continued for the last week. Also, there's been a big change in my energy level. It's gone way up—which probably has a lot to do with finally getting a good night's sleep! But my mood has lifted too. Most of those feelings of anxiety and dread have disappeared, and I can't wait to get going each day. I've had absolutely no side effects from the herb, at least not yet, and I plan to keep taking it for another five or six months, until it's time for my yearly checkup. Then I'll talk to my doctor about whether I should keep taking it. But right now it's doing wonders for me!"

❖

What Are the Symptoms of Menopause?

Any or all of the following symptoms may occur during the various stages of menopause:

- Hot flashes or flushes (best described as intense sensations of heat that spread throughout the body and appear to radiate from the stomach or chest to the face, arms, and legs. Facial skin may redden and profuse sweating may accompany the flash or flush)
- Numbness or tingling in hands and/or feet

- Changes in heart rate (particularly rapid heart beat accompanied by sweating and anxiety; often occurring at night)
- Abdominal bloating
- Breast tenderness
- Weight gain
- Bladder disorders or irritability
- Headaches
- Dizziness
- Insomnia or other sleep disorders
- Severe anxiety
- Mood swings
- Fatigue
- Depression or sadness
- Vaginal dryness, burning, itching, or discomfort

What Are the Causes of Menopausal Symptoms?

Significant decreases in the amounts of estrogen and progesterone circulating in blood and tissues are the primary cause of menopausal symptoms. These hormonal decreases are in turn due to the natural aging of the ovaries and the subsequent decline in ovarian function. Anxiety, stress, poor physical health, emotional problems, and lifestyle factors may all exacerbate the symptoms of menopause.

Menopausal symptoms also may be brought on by the surgical removal of the ovaries.

Conventional Treatments of Menopausal Symptoms

The most common conventional treatment of menopausal symptoms is estrogen replacement therapy (ERT), also called hormone replacement therapy (HRT). Varying strengths of estrogen and progesterone, in tablet and transdermal patch forms, are most frequently prescribed.

Estrogen replacement therapy is an extremely effective treatment and may resolve most menopausal symptoms for many women. Besides providing symptomatic relief for menopause, ERT also provides protection against both heart disease and osteoporosis.

For a substantial number of other women, however, ERT is either contraindicated because of preexisting medical conditions or family medical history, or it is simply not tolerated well because of side effects. Additionally, some clinical research indicates that there is an increased risk of breast and uterine cancer with ERT, so careful patient monitoring is a must, including annual Pap smears and mammograms.

Other women object to being on a potent prescription drug for an indefinite period of time—ERT is often prescribed for many years, if not the rest of a woman's life—and going off ERT often means the resumption of many of the initial symptoms of menopause.

Other conventional treatments for menopausal symptoms include lifestyle counseling and stress-reduction techniques. Calcium supplementation (for prevention of osteporosis) is usually advised. Regular exercise, particularly light weight-bearing exercise, is also recommended both for overall physical and emotional health, to reduce stress, and to strengthen bones.

Using Hypericum to Treat Menopausal Symptoms

As a classic "female tonic," hypericum holds much promise as a treatment for menopausal symptoms. While there is no hard clinical data documenting its effectiveness for this condition, nearly all herbal medicine books and pharmacopoeias—both old and new—list St. John's wort as one of a select group of herbs that are remarkably effective in treating menstrual and menopausal disorders.

Hypericum in particular has wide-ranging treatment applications for the treatment of menopause. For the purely physical symptoms of menopause, it has diuretic, astringent, analgesic, anti-inflammatory, vasorelaxing, and immune-modulating properties. For emotional symptoms and those related to the central nervous system, hypericum has sedating, antidepressant, mood-elevating, and sleep-promoting properties. Before we briefly look at how each of these actions may help relieve the symptoms of menopause, a cautionary note is in order.

The symptoms of menopause are numerous, encompassing, and unique to each woman. Even the highly effective estrogen replacement therapies (ERTs) do not work for all women. And when they do work, it is often only after a long trial period of experimenting with different medications at different dosages. This is also true of alternative treatments for menopause, including herbal therapies. Some herbs work for some women, others don't. Often a combination of herbs, called a herbal formula and prescribed by a herbal medical practitioner, is more effective.

Whatever treatment option is pursued for menopause, maintaining optimal physical health and preventive self-care measures are also more critical than ever at this time.

For these reasons, we offer our suggestions for using hypericum to treat menopausal symptoms with this strong proviso: Please work with a qualified practitioner who is thoroughly knowledgable in women's reproductive health, and let him or her know that you are taking hypericum.

How Hypericum Can Treat Menopausal Symptoms

- **Diuretic and Astringent Action.** Bladder problems, including both frequent and infrequent urination, are frequently symptoms of menopause. Hypericum's diuretic action promotes urination and may help eliminate abdominal bloating and tender or swollen breasts. Its astringent action may help with both frequent urination and excessive sweating.

- **Analgesic Action.** Hypericum has been used effectively to relieve headache pain, nerve pain, and muscle pain. It also may be helpful in relieving the pain of tender and swollen breasts.

- **Anti-inflammatory Action.** Hypericum has clinically proven anti-inflammatory properties that contribute to its pain-relieving action. These anti-inflammatory properties also may help relieve swollen, painful, and stressed tissues and muscles.

- **Vasorelaxing Action.** Hypericum has proven vasorelaxing properties that may help inhibit the arterial constriction that occurs with decreased estrogen levels. This in turn may help relieve irregular or rapid heart beat, profuse sweating, dizziness, and hot flashes or flushes. It may also be a factor in relieving headache pain.

- **Immune-Modulating Action.** Hypericum appears to be a significant immune-modulator. It stimulates the immune system to fight infection and inflammation, and it suppresses or inhibits an overactive immune system (triggered by significantly decreased hormone levels, among other things) that can cause general feelings of physical debilitation. As an immune-modulator, hypericum can both strengthen the body's defenses against infection and relieve inflammation-related pain and discomfort, as well as fatigue and mood changes.

• **Sedating, Antidepressant, Mood-Elevating, and Sleep-Promoting Actions.** There is considerable clinical data documenting hypericum's sedating, anti-anxiety, anti-depressant, and sleep-promoting actions. These in turn may relieve the tension, anxiety, mood changes, and sleep disturbances that are characteristic of menopause.

If you would like to try hypericum for your own meno-pausal symptoms, again we caution you to consult with a qualified medical practitioner—conventional or alternative—and discuss with him or her any preexisting medical conditions you may have or any alternative or conventional medications you are already taking.

You should also review the side effects and contraindications for hypericum listed in Chapter 3. If you have done all that, and you and your practitioner feel comfortable with your taking hypericum, our recommendations for how and when to use it follow.

How and When to Use
Hypericum for Menopausal Symptoms

Start taking hypericum daily. For tablet or capsule form, take 300 mg of hypericum extract 3 times a day with meals, for a total of 900 mg daily. For liquid form, take 1/4 teaspoon (approximately 20 drops) of hypericum extract 3 times a day in a glass of distilled water, with meals, for a total of ³⁄₄ of a teaspoon daily. Both tablet and liquid forms of hypericum should be marked on the label as standarized to 0.3 percent hypericin.

Continue taking hypericum daily for at least two months to see if it effectively relieves your most troubling menopausal symptoms. If you are happy with the way hypericum is working for you, you may continue taking it daily for up to one year, under the supervision of a medical practitioner. For this dosage and duration of treatment, hypericum is exceptionally safe and mild-acting. You and your practitioner might alternately try a regimen of hypericum at lower or higher doses. Clinical studies using hypericum to treat depression, insomnia, and headaches have effectively used dosages ranging from 600 mg to 1,800 mg a day with mild side effects.

If you continue taking hypericum regularly, remember always to advise any medical practitioner of that fact. Of course, stop taking hypericum immediately if you experience any significant side effects.

And When All Else Fails . . .

- Consider taking a hot bath! An excellent, frequently recommended nonmedical treatment for menstrual *and* menopausal discomfort is soaking in a hot tub. We would go further and suggest you try soaking in a hot, steaming tub of hypericum. Therapeutic herbal baths have a long history in traditional medicine, and the skin is an excellent medium for gently absorbing medicines. (Hence the effectiveness of nicotine, nitroglycerin, and estrogen patches.) In fact, you may recall from Chapter 2 that St. John's wort was originally used primarily as a topical agent. The oil or crushed leaves and flowers were applied directly to the skin to heal wounds, prevent infection, reduce inflammation, and treat pain.

If you have access to fresh or dried St. John's wort from a herbal supplier or your garden, wrap 1 to 2 ounces (1 to 2 handfuls) of dried flowers and leaves in cheesecloth or muslin and place in a hot tub. Let the bath water "steep" for about ten minutes, then soak your whole body for at least fifteen to twenty minutes. Try this every night for about one week. You may notice a reduction in muscle pain, breast tenderness, stomach bloating, tension, and vaginal discomfort. Moodiness and poor sleep patterns may also improve. This is a very safe and soothing way to test out the benefits of hypericum for body and soul. (In old herbals, hypericum baths were even recommended for colicky babies!)

• Or savor the pleasures of a restorative tea! For menopausal symptoms in particular, St. John's wort combines wonderfully with several other herbs to form a fine "female tonic" that can relieve anxiety, improve mood, ease hot flashes, promote sleep, and help balance the body's fluctuating hormones. The following tea recipe is both soothing and therapeutic.

St. John's Wort Menopausal Tea
❖

Use dried herbs for this tea recipe.

2 teaspoons St. John's wort
1 teaspoon wild yam
1 teaspoon goldenseal
1 teaspoon valerian
1 teaspoon chamomile
6–7 cups pure spring water, boiled

Place all the dried herb ingredients in a large glass or enameled teapot that you have prewarmed with hot water. (Discard the hot water before adding herbs.) Pour boiling spring water over the herbs, cover the pot, and allow tea to steep for 15 minutes. Strain into a cup or mug and season to taste with honey.

Drink 3 to 4 cups of this tea throughout the day, evenly spaced between meals. You may leave the pot out on your kitchen counter and drink the tea at room temperature. If you prefer your tea hot, gently warm (not boil) the tea in a glass or enameled pot on top of the stove, or stir 1 to 2 teaspoons boiling water into the cup of lukewarm tea. Never microwave herbal tea. Discard any leftover tea and grounds at the end of the day.

CHAPTER 7

❖

Treating Insomnia
with St. John's Wort

The effects of treatment with high doses (300 mg three times daily) of hypericum extract LI 160 on sleep quality and well-being were investigated over a 4-week period. . . . LI 160 induced an increase of deep sleep during the total sleeping period.
—JOURNAL OF GERIATRIC PSYCHIATRY AND NEUROLOGY
OCTOBER 1994, SUPPLEMENT

Insomnia, the most common of several sleep disorders, may affect up to one-third of Americans. Other sleep disorders include sleep apnea (a breathing difficulty that occurs during sleep), restless legs syndrome (discomfort, numbness, or pain in the legs that occurs when an individual is trying to fall asleep), and the very rare narcolepsy (uncontrollable lapses into sleep or extreme drowsiness during waking hours, especially when excited).

Insomnia, sleep apnea, restless legs syndrome, and narcolepsy are collectively known as primary sleep disorders and may occur in the absence of other medical conditions. Secondary sleep disorders, which most frequently involve insomnia, are those that occur as side effects of mental, emotional, or physical illnesses.

Our discussion here focuses only on primary insomnia that appears to be unrelated to other medical conditions and on secondary insomnia that may be the result of conditions such as depression, menopause, or anxiety. In both instances, clinical research indicates that hypericum may be an effective therapeutic aid in promoting deep sleep.

First, however, let's look at the phenomenon of sleep itself.

Defining Sleep

Sleep is a regularly occurring and progressive state of physical inactivity characterized by sleepers' unawareness and unresponsiveness to the physical world, though they can be awakened easily. Individual requirements for sleep vary greatly. Some people function well on as little as five hours of sleep a night. Others need nine to ten hours of sleep to feel rested.

Not all the reasons why we need to sleep are clear, but most scientists believe that the body grows during sleep, especially among the young, and also repairs itself from physical and environmental trauma. Sleep and dreaming also appear to be critical to emotional and mental health, since people who experience both serious sleep deprivation and artificial interruption of dream states may display psychotic behavior.

There are two basic sleep states that regularly alternate with each other throughout the night:

- **Nonrapid eye movement (NREM)** sleep generally involves four progressively deeper and nondreaming stages of sleep (called stages 1 through 4), in which all the physical functions of the body relax and slow down. NREM sleep may be recognized by the fact that the sleeper's eyelids are still. These stages can also be identified when using an electroencephalograph (EEG), a device that measures brain waves.

- **Rapid eye movement (REM)** sleep involves a periodic speeding up of heart rate and breathing, accompanied by rapid eye movements that occur under the eyelids. REM sleep states begin about 1 1/2 hours after NREM sleep starts and occur in progressively longer cycles throughout the night. Early REM states may be as short as 5 minutes, but by the end of the night, toward waking, they may be as long as 30 minutes or more. Since dreaming is believed to occur during REM sleep, this is one reason why we remember our "waking" dreams with such vividness. Infants and young children spend the greatest amount of time in REM sleep. Seniors spend the least. REM sleep is also identified when using an EEG.

A good night's sleep is generally defined as one where we experience the full four states of increasingly deeper NREM sleep with regularly occurring and progressively longer stages of REM sleep. When this happens, we easily fall asleep and stay asleep, wake up naturally and on time, and feel physically and mentally renewed. When this doesn't occur on a regular basis, we join the large and growing roster of insomniacs.

Defining Insomnia

Insomnia is generally defined as poor or inadequate sleep and may include any or all of the following symptoms: difficulty falling asleep; inability to sleep through the night; waking up too early; waking up sporadically throughout the night; not sleeping deeply enough (restless sleep); waking up feeling tired.

The physical symptoms of insomnia, beyond those that relate directly to nightly sleep patterns, may considerably impact family and work life. They include fatigue and drowsiness, anxiety and irritability, a need to sleep during the day ("nap"), poor concentration, and impaired memory.

There are three basic types of insomnia:

- **Transient insomnia** refers to poor or inadequate sleep that persists for only a few nights. Transient insomnia is self-resolving and generally requires no therapeutic treatment, conventional or alternative.

- **Short-term insomnia** refers to poor or inadequate sleep that lasts for up to three weeks. Short-term insomnia that progresses beyond a week may require some therapeutic treatment, conventional or alternative.

- **Chronic insomnia** refers to poor or inadequate sleep that persists for three weeks or longer. Chronic insomnia takes an enormous physical and mental toll and requires therapeutic treatment.

Conventional Treatments of Insomnia

Conventional treatments of insomnia run the gamut from homespun advice (take warm baths, drink warm milk, count sheep) to lifestyle counseling (avoid caffeine and nicotine, exercise regularly) to pharmaceutical intervention (stimulants for daytime fatigue, hypnotics and sedatives to produce an artificial sleep).

Some of the homespun advice works on a limited basis for short-term insomnia. Lifestyle changes improve overall health in the long term, which may be enough to resolve sleeping problems.

Prescription drugs, whether stimulants or hypnotics, should be viewed as very limited short-term treatment reserved for severe cases of insomnia. If possible, avoid both types of drugs. They are very addictive, require increasingly larger doses to be effective, and actually decrease good sleep in the long run by significantly reducing REM stages (when dreaming occurs).

Using Hypericum to Treat Insomnia

A long-respected nervine and tonic in traditional herbal medicines, St. John's wort has the dual therapeutic effect of being both gently sedating and mildly energizing. These therapeutic effects aren't contradictions in terms. All the great herbal tonics share these complementary properties. By strengthening and balancing weak or injured organ systems and biochemical processes, tonics enhance general physical well-being, reduce fatigue, and increase energy. Physical well-being in turn counteracts tension, stress, and anxiety, and promotes good sleep.

We also know from our discussion of hypericum and depression in Chapter 5 that there is substantial clinical evidence of hypericum's effectiveness in treating some of the physical debilitation, fatigue, anxiety, and sleep problems associated with mild-to-moderate depression.

At least one clinical study also has specifically looked at hypericum as a sleep aid in twelve healthy and older volunteers. It found a measurable increase in deep sleep over the whole sleeping period that was consistently observable (using EEG) in stages 3 and 4 of NREM sleep. This study used the LI 160 hypericum formulation (300 mg standardized to 0.3% hypericin, 3 times a day), for four weeks.

Several other studies have focused on hypericum's general effect on EEG-recorded brain wave activity in depressed patients and noted increases in theta waves (those associated with sleep and deep meditation). Further, hypericum didn't decrease alertness and clarity, as did one of the prescription sedatives to which it was compared.

HOW TO USE HYPERICUM TO TREAT INSOMNIA

Again, we strongly advise you to work with a qualified practitioner if you are going to try hypericum for your insomnia. If you have chronic insomnia, it's also important to have a thorough physical checkup and rule out any other physical problems. This is especially important if there is any chance that your insomnia is a symptom of an underlying depression. In such a case, it's critical that you treat the depression first, which requires a more potent dosage of hypericum and a longer treatment time. (The insomnia will probably resolve itself during treatment.)

❖

Brian's Story:
Finding Relief During Recovery

Brian, a small-town contractor who renovates landmark houses in southern New England, had always been skeptical about anything "weird or new-agey," especially when it came to his health. He believed in a conservative approach to health care and in tried-and-true conventional medicine. And if all else failed, Brian advocated a stoic "live-with-it" attitude toward pain and bad health.

Then a fall from a ladder on a job site eighteen months ago left him with torn muscles, chronic back pain, and the threat of losing not only his livelihood but his peace of mind. Worst of all, conventional medicine failed him. Heat packs and whirlpool baths provided only temporary relief from his pain. Prescription

painkillers—when they had any effect—left him nause-
ated, groggy, and unable to work. After eight months of
trying to live with pain and disability, Brian had also
become mildly depressed and an insomniac. He was
ready to throw in the towel and turn his business over
to his grown son. But his daughter-in-law offered him a
"last resort" option. She knew of an acupuncturist in
the northern part of the state who practiced traditional
Chinese medicine. This man had used acupuncture and
acupressure to successfully treat a friend of hers with
chronic back pain.

Despite an innate resistance to anything "different,"
Brian was desperate enough to give this alternative practitioner a try. After just two weeks of acupuncture and
acupressure treatments, Brian began to experience the
first significant relief of pain in almost a year. While this
thrilled him and should have been enough (Brian
thought) to shake off the moodiness, depressed feelings,
and recurrent bouts of insomnia that he had also been
experiencing, it wasn't. He was almost pain free, but he
was still unhappy. Reluctantly, Brian talked about these
problems with his new practitioner, whom he had come
to trust and regard as a friend. Much to Brian's surprise,
the doctor told him he was suffering from depression.
And he recommended an herb to treat it—St. John's
wort. Brian, a dyed-in-the-wool swamp Yankee who had
eschewed even aspirin for most of his life, began taking
300 mg of St. John's wort three times a day with meals.
And now he's a vocal advocate of the herb's effectiveness.

"I've been taking St. John's wort for about six
months now for what my doctor calls 'mild depression'
and for my insomnia, both of which I think were due to
all the stress from worrying about not being able to
work again. I'm only fifty-eight. I have to say, I was a

little nervous about taking a herb. But I've been very happy with the results. It's eliminated all the symptoms of my depression, that 'blue' feeling that I just couldn't seem to shake. And I have no trouble with insomnia anymore. After I had been taking it for about two weeks, I began sleeping through the night for the first time in almost a year. You can't imagine how wonderful that felt after being just plain bone tired, every day, day after day. I haven't had any negative side effects so far, although my doctor told me to be careful about sun exposure. And I was, since I work outdoors most of the time. During the summer, when I was taking St. John's wort, I was working on the exterior of a house for over two months. But I used a sunscreen, and I had no problems with sunburn. I'm so glad I found St. John's wort, and I plan to take it as long as I need it."

❖

For Short-Term Insomnia—

We recommend that you try hypericum for 1 to 2 weeks in *tea form*, traditionally called an infusion. Traditional practitioners recommend this therapeutic form of taking herbs most often. We provide a basic recipe for making St. John's wort tea in Chapter 4. For a tea that has more sedating properties, you may want to try the recipe for St. John's Wort Insomnia Tea provided at the end of this chapter. If your insomnia does not resolve itself after two weeks, try our suggestions for treating chronic insomnia.

For Chronic Insomnia—

We suggest you follow the treatment plan used in the sleep study with healthy volunteers (described above). In this case, you can use tablets, capsules, or liquid extract as follows:

Tablet or Capsule Forms: 300 mg of hypericum extract standardized to 0.3 percent hypericin, 3 times a day with meals, for a total of 900 mg daily. Take it for 4 weeks, then stop. If insomnia has been resolved, switch to St. John's Wort Tea (Chapter 4) as a maintenance plan. Have 1 cup after dinner, and 1 cup an hour before retiring. If insomnia returns, see a practitioner.

Liquid Extract Form: 1/4 teaspoon (approximately 20 drops) of hypericum extract standardized to 0.3 percent hypericin, 3 times a day in distilled water, with meals, for a total of 3/4 teaspoon daily. Take it for 4 weeks, then stop. If insomnia has been resolved, switch to St. John's Wort Tea (Chapter 4) as a maintenance plan. Have 1 cup after dinner, and 1 cup an hour before retiring. If insomnia returns, see a practitioner.

St. John's Wort Insomnia Tea

❖

Use dried herbs for this tea recipe.

  2 teaspoons St. John's wort
  1 teaspoon hops
  1 teaspoon valerian
  1 teaspoon chamomile
  4–6 cups pure spring water, boiled

Place all the dried herb ingredients in a large glass or enameled teapot that you have prewarmed with hot water. (Discard the hot water before adding herbs.) Pour boiling spring water over the herbs, cover the pot, and allow tea to steep for 15 minutes. Strain into a cup or mug and season to taste with honey.

Drink 3 to 4 cups of this tea throughout the day, evenly spaced between meals. You may leave the pot out on your kitchen counter and drink the tea at room temperature. If you prefer your tea hot, gently warm (not boil) the tea in a glass or enameled pot on top of the stove, or stir 1 to 2 teaspoons boiling water into the cup of lukewarm tea. Never microwave herbal tea. Discard any leftover tea and grounds at the end of the day.

CHAPTER 8

❖

Fighting Viruses and Strengthening Immunity with St. John's Wort

Following attachment and entry of human immunodeficiency virus (HIV) into a host cell, the HIV genomic RNA is reverse transcribed to cDNA. This step may be inhibited by hypericin, a compound that induces alterations of the retroviral capsid. Incubation of HIV with hypericin rendered the virus noninfectious. The replication of HIV was blocked early; HIV cDNA could not be detected in cells challenged with hypericin-treated HIV.
—AIDS RESEARCH AND HUMAN RETROVIRUSES,
NOVEMBER 1992, SUPPLEMENT

Among all the recent news about St. John's wort, perhaps none is more dramatic and exciting than that of its extraordinary antiviral properties.

Especially in the last ten years, virologists (those who study viruses) have focused their research on the therapeutic action of the two most chemically active constituents found in St. John's wort: hypericin and pseudohypericin. What they have found is astonishing: a potential multipurpose antiviral agent with the ability to disable some of the most powerful human viruses known to science.

First, Just What Are Viruses?

A virus is a microscopic infectious organism that comprises a core of nucleic acid (which contains the virus's

DNA or RNA), surrounded by a coat of protein. It is this protein coat that floods the bloodstream with antibodies specific to the virus, signaling in blood tests that an infection is or was present.

Viruses are grouped according to the type of nucleic acid they have at their core and also by their appearance. There are thousands of viruses, but among the major ones that cause infections in humans are the herpesviruses (herpes simplex I and II, mononucleosis, chicken pox, shingles, Epstein-Barr), the adenoviruses (conjunctivitis and upper respiratory infections), the rhinoviruses (common cold), the myxoviruses (flu or influenza), and the retroviruses (AIDS).

Unlike bacteria, which are large, living organisms that can exist throughout the body and produce toxins, viruses are tiny, nonliving organisms that cannot exert any effect or even survive without first inhabiting a host cell. They usually enter the body through the respiratory tract, but also can enter in blood and other fluids through body orifices and cuts in the skin. Some viruses are also passed from mother to child during pregnancy or childbirth.

Once in the body, viruses take up residence in a host cell. There they may kill the cell, transform or mutate it—thereby wreaking havoc throughout the body—or simply lie dormant for years, as does HIV, the virus that causes AIDS.

The body's natural viral-fighting defense mechanism is the powerful immune system. Stimulated by the presence of the first virus-infected cells in the body, the immune system produces interferons, protein substances that travel to healthy cells in the body and make them resistant to further infection by the original virus.

Unfortunately, there are few artificial agents that mimic the powerful antiviral action of the body's immune system.

In contrast to the wide range of antibiotics available to treat bacterial infections, there are only a handful of pharmaceutical drugs that effectively target viruses.

However, that situation may be about to change.

Hypericum As Virus Fighter

In laboratory studies over the last ten years, researchers have discovered that both hypericin and pseudohypericin, two of the most active chemical constituents found in St. John's wort, possess powerful antiviral action against many viruses, including:

- Influenza A and B
- Herpes Simplex I and II
- Epstein-Barr
- Vesicular Stomatitis
- Equine Infectious Anemia
- Hepatitis C
- HIV (Human Immune Deficiency Virus)

Hypericin, in particular, has demonstrated potent antiviral capabilities. Studies of hypericin's properties, using synthetic versions of the chemical, have revealed two antiviral mechanisms. Like the body's natural interferons, hypericin protects healthy cells from invasion and infection when a virus enters the body. But hypericin has another extraordinary action: it literally inactivates the virus, stopping it in its tracks. As of this date, researchers still don't understand *how* hypericin does that, but a plethora of research investigations are presently under way to unravel the mystery.

Hypericum As an Immune-Stimulator and -Modulator

Hypericin and pseudohypericin also have documented immune-stimulating and immune-modulating properties. As discussed in Chapter 5, these particular therapeutic properties of St. John's wort may be partly responsible for its success as an antidepressant.

Depression has a known physical component—an excess production of interleukins that debilitates the body overall and makes a person more prone to infection. St. John's wort is believed to help slow down excessive interleukin production and simultaneously balance and strengthen an overworked immune system. When people take St. John's wort for depression, their physical symptoms are often the first to go. In one of our personal stories (see Chapter 5), a health and science writer who began using St. John's wort to treat her major depression also noticed, about six months into treatment, that her chronic and debilitating bouts with colds, bronchitis, and pneumonia had completely disappeared!

Clearly, the therapeutic potential of a plant botanical that combines specific antiviral action with immune-modulating properties is enormous. As we go to press, multiple patient studies are under way using hypericin to treat AIDS, hepatitis, and various viral skin infections. More studies are planned. Whether St. John's wort fulfills its potential as a near-miraculous antiviral remains to be seen, but the signs are more than promising.

In the meantime, should we use St. John's wort to treat our own everyday viruses, such as the common colds and seasonal flus that arrive like clockwork every autumn? The answer is a tempered "yes."

Using Hypericum to Fight Your Viruses and Strengthen Immunity

We don't recommend using St. John's wort on your own to self-treat AIDS or hepatitis, unless you are working closely with a medical practitioner who specializes in these viruses. And we also caution you to remember that the results obtained in small, controlled clinical studies with synthetic versions of a plant's chemicals may not be easily replicated at home.

With those provisos, we do believe St. John's wort may be helpful in preventing colds and flus—or at least lessening their effects—as part of a self-care regimen that also includes good nutrition and vitamin supplements, particularly vitamin C, and other immune-enhancing herbs, such as echinacea.

To Help Prevent or Lessen the Effects of Colds and Flus

First of all, we don't recommend taking St. John's wort year-round as a preventive, unless, of course, you are being treated for depression. We also don't recommend taking it at depression-level strength (300 mg, 3 times a day) either. There is no clinical evidence that St. John's wort has a cumulative antiviral effect, though we are aware that it is used as a daily tonic in some European countries. Even the old herbal books don't recommend St. John's wort as an everyday restorative or tonic, as they sometimes do for ginger and echinacea.

However, if you'd like to try St. John's wort as a short-term preventive for colds and flus, we suggest you start taking it at the beginning of the cold season, usually in early autumn, and continue taking it until the start of spring.

Instead of using tablets, capsules, or liquid extracts (though tablets and capsules come in dosages as low as 100 mg), we recommend that you take St. John's wort as a tea or infusion made from the dried herb. (See Chapter 4 for the basic St. John's Wort Tea recipe.) The tea is a gentler, but still potent, form of the herb, and using the whole plant in dried herb form gives you a full complement of all the herb's beneficial chemical constituents.

It's also easier to add more "cold specific" herbs to the tea, ones that relieve your symptoms naturally, in the event that you do get a cold or flu. For instance, if you come down with a cold, you might want to add one or more of the following dried herbs to your basic St. John's wort recipe:

- a teaspoon of rosehips (for extra Vitamin C)
- a teaspoon of peppermint (as a decongestant)
- a teaspoon of echinacea (to fight associated bacterial infections)
- a teaspoon of goldenseal (to help break up phlegm).

Remember to add 1 cup (8 ounces) of distilled spring water to the pot for every extra teaspoon of dried herbs you use.

Let's move on to our last treatment chapter and a look at one of the most innovative new uses for St. John's wort—as a weight loss aid!

CHAPTER 9

❖

Achieving Weight Loss
with St. John's Wort

(With regard to weight loss) St. John's wort appears to interrupt the depression-binge-resolution cycle by helping improve mood.
—FROM A POSTER PRESENTATION AT THE ANNUAL
NORTH AMERICAN ASSOCIATION FOR
OBESITY CONFERENCE, 1997

None of the older herbal books—or, for that matter, any of the fine newer ones—mentions St. John's wort as a treatment for obesity or as a weight loss aid. Of course, old-time traditional healers and their patients were vastly more concerned about surviving the exigencies of medieval life—demons, despotic rulers, burnings at stakes, plagues, poverty, incessant warfare with exceedingly sharp weapons—than they were about losing fat. Indeed, they needed all the fat they could get.

Only modern man and woman could turn the shedding of an extra 15 pounds into a near-religious mania. It's no surprise, then, that the commercial herbal manufacturing industry would jump on the weight loss bandwagon and begin marketing "natural" herbal products designed to help lose weight.

And they were aided immeasurably in their efforts when American Home Products had to withdraw its fabulously successful multibillion-dollar prescription diet drug, Redux, from the marketplace because it caused potentially fatal heart-valve problems. Soon a flood of highly touted "herbal phen-fens" appeared, several with St. John's wort in them. But did they really work? And were they really safe?

At least one of those herbal weight loss products received a good deal of bad press. It combined St. John's wort with the potent herbal stimulant ephedra (mahuang), which can be potentially fatal for people with heart problems. Conventional doctors, now deprived of a powerful prescription diet drug, were also roundly scornful of herbal weight loss products, viewing them as not much more than silly placebos for the desperate and foolish.

Obesity is no laughing matter. Being chronically overweight by twenty pounds or more has been directly and indirectly linked to the three greatest killers of the late twentieth century: diabetes, heart disease, and cancer. And then there are the enormous emotional and social tolls to pay for being fat in a society that deifies being thin. A safe and effective natural weight-loss aid is sorely needed. And St. John's wort may partly answer that need.

❖

Todd's Story:
Beating the Munchies the Easy Way

Todd, a forty-year-old computer salesman, didn't immediately notice that his appetite had changed and that he was slowly but surely losing weight.

"I had been taking St. John's wort for depression for almost eight months when I first realized that my appetite had decreased significantly and I was losing weight. More than that, I didn't crave certain junk foods or sweets anymore. And when I did eat, I got full very quickly, so I ate less at meals.

"I didn't really need to lose weight, but over the course of just a month or so, I lost about five to seven pounds. The effects would probably be even greater for someone who is really overweight and has more pounds to lose. I even lost weight over the Christmas holidays! That's incredible, because I usually go nuts for food during the holidays. But not only wasn't I very hungry at the big holiday dinners, but sweets and desserts, which I couldn't get enough of before, simply didn't appeal to me.

"This decrease and change in appetite was very subtle. I didn't even begin to realize it was happening until I had been on St. John's wort for many months.

"Recently, I had to stop taking St. John's wort for a month. Within a few days I noticed a significant increase in my appetite, plus my cravings for junk food were back. I plan to go back on St. John's wort as soon as I can."

❖

Why St. John's Wort May Work for Weight Loss

There are at least three centuries-old traditional uses of St. John's wort that point to its potential as a useful weight loss aid: it is an excellent diuretic; it elevates mood by relieving anxiety; and it has mildly energizing properties, largely due to its tonic effect. All three of those actions can go a long way to supporting a solid weight-loss plan that also includes a low-fat diet and exercise.

Among the nondepressed, eating in response to anxiety and stress is an all too common phenomenon. But recent research indicates that it may be as an antidepressant that St. John's wort is most potent in helping people to lose weight. Eating disorders, including binge eating, are among the key symptoms of major depression, and many of those symptoms were alleviated in the clinical trials that tested St. John's wort as an antidepressant. Prozac, the serotonin reuptake inhibitor that St. John's wort most closely resembles, is also associated with weight loss.

The depression-weight loss angle soon became the focus of serious attention. In fact, as we finish this book, the New York Obesity Research Center, a conglomerate of scientists from St. Luke's-Roosevelt Hospital, Columbia University, Rockefeller University, and Cornell University, has just completed their first patient study of St. John's wort and weight loss, and has another larger, double-blind, and placebo-controlled study scheduled for 1998. While the results of their first study would not be published until 1998, researchers were able to present some preliminary findings at the fall 1997 annual meeting of the North American Association for Obesity in Cancún, Mexico.

According to their findings, St. John's wort may be a significant weight-loss aid because, by improving mood, it interrupts the "depression-binge-resolution cycle." In other words, by stabilizing mood, it mitigates the tendency of depressed or anxious people to begin overeating again. The "losing weight, facing a crisis, overeating in response, and gaining back weight syndrome" is common in overeaters, as it is in others who use substances of abuse as mood changers (smokers and alcoholics, for instance).

The St. John's wort product used in the Obesity Research Center's study was Herbal Phen Fuel, from Twin Laboratories in Ronkonkoma, New York. Sold in capsule form, Twin Lab's formulation contains 325 mg of hypericum, standardized to 0.3% hypericin. At 3 capsules a day, that amount of hypericum actually exceeds the recommended daily dose for mild-to-moderate depression. So it is not surprising that the same changes in eating behavior observed in depression studies might also occur with a product like Herbal Phen Fuel.

In addition, Herbal Phen Fuel is combined with another herb, *Citrus auranticum* (orange bitter), a mild stimulant long used in Chinese herbal medicine and considered a safer alternative to mahuang (ephedra). This clearly stimulating herb also contributes to the product's weight-loss effects. It also contains small amounts of green tea, ginger, and cayenne.

❖

Magda's Story: A Sweet—and Trim—Tale

Magda, a fifty-two-year-old freelance writer who had been unsuccessfully dieting for years, had an experience similar to Sarah's (see Chapter 3) and naturally lost weight after she began taking St. John's wort for her lifelong mild depressive symptoms.

"Since I started taking St. John's wort a little over a year ago, my weight has dropped over twenty pounds, slowly but surely. I'm one of those people who's been slightly depressed all her life, and I think that had a lot to do with the fact that I also became a compulsive overeater. It seemed like I thought about food and eating all day long, and then in the evening I'd binge on sweets on top of overeating during the day.

"All that compulsive behavior's disappeared since I started taking St. John's wort. Most of the time now, I eat only when I'm hungry, and I eat less and eat better. This is something that seems to have happened so naturally that I still haven't gotten used to not buying cartons of 'goodies' every time I shop, especially ice cream and cookies. In fact, last night I threw out a couple of cartons of ice cream that had freezer burn! It's not that I don't like sweets anymore. I'll still have a couple of cookies, a piece of cake, or a dish of ice cream now and then, but usually only after a meal and for dessert. Before I started taking St. John's wort, I'd eat a whole box of cookies in one evening, just watching television."

❖

Should You Use St. John's Wort for Weight Loss?

We think a good deal more research is needed into the potential weight-loss properties of St. John's wort, particularly when it is combined with other herbs.

The most successful weight-loss programs are always long-term and multidimensional. A low-fat but ample diet, regular daily exercise, behavior modification, and losing weight at a small but steady rate over many months—these are the key ingredients to a successful weight-loss plan. Despite its safety, we never recommend taking St. John's wort at high doses for a long time, especially if you're not depressed.

On the other hand, if you have a good weight-loss program already in place, and need some additional supportive therapy—particularly for anxiety or irritability—we see no reason not to use St. John's wort as a tea (infusion) on a daily basis. You may use our basic recipe (Chapter 4), or try the St. John's Wort Menopausal Tea (Chapter 6, and our apologies to the men among you), but eliminate the wild yam (that's the herb with the most "natural" estrogen).

Let's move on to our last chapter to take a look at where St. John's wort is heading.

PART III

❖

Future Possibilities
with St. John's Wort

CHAPTER 10

❖

Looking Ahead

Hypericin has been reported to inhibit the growth of glioma cell lines in vitro and to be a potent inducer of glioma cell death due to inhibition of protein kinase C (PKC). . . . In this regard the glioma inhibitory activity is reported to be equal to or greater than Tamoxifen.
—AMERICAN HERBAL PHARMACOPOEIA™
ST. JOHN'S WORT MONOGRAPH
JULY 1997

As we move into the twenty-first century, what new developments can we expect in the use of St. John's wort to treat illness and disease?

We believe researchers will focus primarily on the therapeutic potential of St. John's wort in treating cancer, myriad viruses, particularly AIDS and hepatitis, and major depression. Research will no doubt continue into some of the lesser known—or less celebrated—therapeutic properties of St. John's wort, including its possible effectiveness in treating heart disease, several disorders of childhood, among them enuresis (bed-wetting) and attention deficit disorder (ADD), chronic headache, and alcoholism. We also expect that St. John's wort will become more widely used as a "female tonic," particularly for the symptoms of menopause when used in combination with other plant herbs.

Let's briefly look at some of the major potential uses of St. John's wort.

ST. JOHN'S WORT: AN ANTICANCER MEDICINE

The reported ability of St. John's wort to treat glioma (see the start of this chapter), a particularly malignant and inoperable form of brain cancer, was later verified in one human patient. There it proved to be more effective than Tamoxifen, the standard chemotherapy drug of choice. The enzyme protein kinase C (PKC), which helps regulate cell growth and cell mutation rates, is found in higher quantities in the body when certain cancers are present. In some cases, inhibiting PKC activity, which is what the hypericin in St. John's wort does, can also inhibit the growth of cancerous tumors.

Currently, several studies are under way to investigate the effectiveness of hypericin in treating breast cancer and melanoma (the most malignant form of skin cancer). Also under investigation is its ability to inhibit excessive subretinal cell growth in certain eye conditions.

In addition to its direct anticancer properties, the hypericin in St. John's wort, a photosensitive plant herb, is also being investigated as a combination cancer treatment with laser therapy. Laser-activated hypericin significantly inactivated human carcinoma, sarcoma, and melanoma cells in laboratory studies; limited research in human patients will follow. In fact, hypericin's antiviral properties are significantly enhanced in the presence of light.

ST. JOHN'S WORT: AN ANTIVIRAL MEDICINE

As we discussed in Chapters 2 and 8, hypericin—the most chemically active constituent found in St. John's wort—has exhibited powerful antiviral effects in laboratory studies and in human studies.

Hypericin is particularly potent in treating what are known as lipid-enveloped viruses (in which a thin covering of a fat-like substance surrounds the virus's outer protein layer) and the retroviruses (RNA-containing viruses that transform themselves into DNA when they enter a host cell, with dire consequences). The most well-known lipid-enveloped viruses are hepatitis, herpes simplex, and influenza. HIV and AIDS are the most prevalent retroviruses.

In the next few years we will see more frequent and large-scale studies of patients using hypericin to treat AIDS and hepatitis. Right now, several small ones are already in progress throughout the country. We may also expect to see human studies of hypericin's effectiveness, taken internally and applied topically, for the herpes simplex and papilloma (wart) viruses.

St. John's Wort as an Immune-Modulator

Complementing its superior antiviral properties is the considerable immunotropic action found in St. John's wort. It stimulates the immune system in the presence of infection or debilitation, and it inhibits an overactive immune system that has been taxed by chronic disease or stress.

We may expect to see St. John's wort take a more prominent place as a preventive tonic against everyday colds and flus, much the way echinacea has been used by the general public for the last several years. However, St. John's wort may be a milder immune-modulator than echinacea, which is not recommended for people with serious immune-related diseases (such as AIDS and lupus).

ST. JOHN'S WORT:
AN ANTIDEPRESSANT MEDICINE

The single greatest application of St. John's wort will no doubt be in the treatment of depression. A substantial body of clinical research, together with nearly twenty years' worth of successful use in millions of German patients, leaves little doubt that St. John's wort is a very effective and safe treatment for mild-to-moderate depression.

Soon the National Institutes of Health and Office of Alternative Medicine will begin a multimillion-dollar, multicenter study of hypericum's effectiveness in treating depressed patients throughout the United States. In a few years, when the results of that study are in—barring any unforeseen problems with heretofore unknown side effects—we can expect the FDA to approve St. John's wort as an antidepressant. With that approval will come FDA regulation, the ramifications of which are not clear. St. John's wort may be available only through a doctor's prescription. And if the pharmaceutical industry steps in to act as "mediator," we can surely expect to see the costs for St. John's wort skyrocket.

Until then, more and more people will use St. John's wort on their own—hopefully in concert with a medical practitioner—to treat depression, seasonal affective disorder (SAD), anxiety, insomnia, headache pain, and simple tension.

❖

Harry's Story:
Overcoming Uncontrollable Pain

St. John's wort has long been used by alternative medical practitioners to treat chronic pain of the muscles and nerves. Currently, many people are using St. John's wort to treat the chronic pain of fibromyalgia, an old disease that has recently become more widely diagnosed. Estimated to affect over ten million people, fibromyalgia (also known as fibrositis or myofascial pain syndrome) is chronic and debilitating musculoskeletal pain throughout the body, but especially in the back, neck, and shoulders. It is often accompanied by sleep disorders and extreme fatigue. Recent research indicates that fibromyalgia may in part be caused by low levels of serotonin in the body, and the most current treatments have included both painkillers and antidepressants that raise serotonin levels, such as Prozac—though the disease isn't necessarily related to depression.

St. John's wort, with its triple therapeutic action of relieving pain, promoting sleep, and increasing serotonin levels, has worked remarkably well for many people who suffer from fibromyalgia, including Harry, a forty-six-year-old high school teacher.

"I have had fibromyalgia for almost four years now, and it's particularly bad during the cold winter months. Being on my feet teaching all day made it even worse. I'd become dependent on painkillers to get through the school year, and I had also tried several prescription antidepressants. But nothing was really working.

"Last year I joined a chronic-pain support group, and one of the members remarked that she'd been experiencing some real relief from her 'fibro' by taking St. John's wort. It not only helped her pain, but she was also sleeping better. I decided to give it a try, and on her recommendation, I began taking three hundred milligrams, three times a day. It's been seven months since I started taking the St. John's wort, and I've never felt as good! For the first time in four years my fibromyalgia seems to be under control. In fact, I've just gone through my first winter on St. John's wort, and I've barely had to touch my painkillers. Plus I sleep through the night almost all the time now, and that was very rare for me before. I have to say that I did have some stomach upset and nausea when I first started taking St. John's wort, but that went away in a month or two. And the tradeoff was more than worth it. St. John's is the best thing that's happened to me in years!"

❖

OTHER MEDICINAL USES OF ST. JOHN'S WORT

Below are several of the lesser-known, or less-understood, therapeutic applications of St. John's wort, both anecdotal and scientific. We expect interest and research into these applications to increase dramatically in the next few years.

- **PMS, Menstrual and Menopausal Problems.** St. John's wort has a long history as a "female" tonic, largely overlooked amid the current excitement about its antidepressant and antiviral properties. We expect that situation to change. As we discussed in great detail in Chapter 6, St. John's wort is a superior analgesic (relieves pain), antispasmodic (relieves muscle cramping), diuretic (alleviates excess fluids), sleep promoter, and anti-anxiety medicine. All these properties make it a superlative treatment for the commonly caused symptoms of PMS, menstrual discomfort, and menopause.

- **Children's Disorders: Enuresis and Attention Deficit Disorder.** St. John's wort has long been used successfully to treat bed-wetting (enuresis) in children. Usually the child is given St. John's wort in tea (dried herb form) or in a tincture (liquid extract form) an hour or so before retiring for the night. Often the bed-wetting problem is resolved within a week. (St. John's wort, in this same manner, also has been used to treat children's nightmares and night terrors.)

In this book, we don't recommend giving St. John's wort to children in general, and so we have provided no dosing information for this indication of the herb. However, if this is a problem for you and your child, we heartily recommend you see a qualified herbal practitioner.

Currently, there is also much anecdotal information about the effectiveness of St. John's wort in treating attention deficit disorder (ADD). Subscribers at several of the better herbal medicine sites on the Internet indicate they are using St. John's wort, in tea or liquid extract form, to treat their children's ADD successfully. Clearly, some of the herb's powerful antidepressant properties are operative here, as well as its ability to relieve stress and promote deep sleep. Expect to see further developments in this area.

- **Alcoholism and Gastrointestinal Illnesses Associated with Alcoholism.** At least one study involving 57 patients with alcoholism and associated chronic digestive illnesses (Krylov and Ivatov in *Lik Sprave*, 1993; article in Russian), demonstrated that St. John's wort relieved not only the depressive symptoms of the alcohol addiction, but also the stomach problems. Patients received St. John's wort in infusion (tea) form, four to five times a day for two months. They also received psychotherapy.

With regard to treating the alcoholism itself, we do

know from the very preliminary studies of St. John's wort and obesity that there is a component in the plant herb that appears to interrupt the "craving-binge" mechanism of addiction.

In the above instance, it may be difficult to assess the effects of St. John's wort in treating the gastrointestinal complaints: just stopping drinking is enough to relieve some people's associated stomach problems, particularly gastritis. However, St. John's wort does have a long and successful history of treating other stomach and intestinal ailments, most notably stomach cramping and pain, as well as diarrhea.

• **Pain Relief.** St. John's wort is noted for its analgesic properties. It relieves painful stomach cramping and also has been used to treat chronic headache. It is especially esteemed by herbalists for its significant relief of the pain associated with nerve illnesses; shingles is an excellent example of such pain. Expect to see St. John's wort appear more frequently in topical form for just this purpose.

• **Antibiotic and Antibacterial.** First and foremost, St. John's wort has been renowned for its wound-healing action. Again, we would expect to see more topical forms of St. John's wort appear on the market for home first-aid treatment.

One of the earliest uses of St. John's wort was to fight bacterial infections. In fact, it was used to treat malaria in the Middle Ages. Currently, scientists are investigating its effectiveness in treating tuberculosis, which has made a strong comeback in the late twentieth century, and in helping eradicate the increasingly prevalent epidemics of staph infection, many of which are resistant to conventional antibiotics.

- **Heart Disease.** Some of the latest clinical research into the chemical constituents of St. John's wort indicate that at least one constituent, proanthocyanidin, may protect the heart against coronary vasospasm. Vasospasm is what happens, for instance, during an angina attack. The coronary arteries drastically narrow, blood flow to the heart is restricted, severe chest pain follows, and the risk of heart attack dramatically rises. In a 1991 laboratory study, proanthocyanidin extracted from St. John's wort significantly relaxed coronary arteries isolated from animals (much the way nitroglycerin does in an angina attack). Clearly this is an area where we can expect to see more research conducted.

In the last twenty-five years, as alternative medicine has slowly but steadily made inroads into mainstream medicine, no other plant herb has received the popular attention, scientific scrutiny, and begrudging respect that St. John's wort has in just the last few years. The therapeutic applications of what many considered just a nuisance weed seem unlimited right now.

The healing gifts of St. John's wort are, of course, immeasurable. But so, too, is the bridge it spans from alternative to conventional medicine. At long last those traditionally opposing camps now seem ready to shake hands, amazingly enough, over the sun-kissed blossoms of a weed that midsummer revelers once tossed into bonfires to chase away demons. The story is just beginning.

Appendix: Suppliers, Resources, and Organizations

I. HERB SUPPLIERS—MAIL, PHONE, AND FAX ORDERS

The following companies sell herbal **liquid extracts, tablets, capsules,** and **dried herbs**. Write, phone, or fax for product and ordering information.

Blessed Herbs
109 Barre Plains Road
Oakham, MA 01068
Tel: 508-882-3839
Fax: 508-882-3755

Eclectic Institute
14385 SE Lusted Road
Sandy, OR 97055-9549
Tel: 800-332-4372
Fax: 503-668-3227

Elixer Tonics & Teas
8612 Melrose Avenue
West Hollywood, CA 90069
Tel: 888-4TONICS

Frontier Herbs
Box 299
Norway, IA 52318
Tel: 800-669-3275
Fax: 319-227-7966

Gaia Herbs
108 Island Ford Road
Brevard, NC 28712
Tel: 800-831-7780
Fax: 800-717-1722

Herb Pharm
20260 Williams Highway
Williams, OR 97544
Tel: 800-348-4372
Fax: 800-545-7392

Hickey Chemists
888 Second Avenue
New York, NY 10017
Tel: 800-724-5566

Hypericum Buyers Club
8205 Santa Monica
Boulevard
Los Angeles, CA 90068
Tel: 888-497-3742

Indiana Botanic Gardeners
P.O. Box 5
Hammond, IN 46325
Tel: 219-947-4040

McZand Herbal
P.O. Box 5312
Santa Monica, CA 90409
Tel: 310-822-0500
Fax: 310-822-1050

Merz Apothecary
4716 N. Lincoln Avenue
Chicago, IL 60625
Tel: 773-989-0900/
800-252-0275
Fax: 773-989-8108

Nature's Plus
548 Broadhollow Road
Melville, NY 11747
Tel: 800-645-9500
Fax: 516-249-2022

NatureWorks
207 East 94th Street
New York, NY 10128
Tel: 800-226-6227
Fax: 212-860-8323

Nutrition Headquarters, Inc.
One Nutrition Plaza
Carbondale, IL 62901-8825
Tel: 618-457-8100
Fax: 618-529-4533

Pacific Botanicals
4350 Fish Hatchery Road
Grants Pass, OR 97527
Tel: 541-479-7777
Fax: 541-479-5271

Planetary Formulations
P.O. Box 533
Soquel, CA 95073
Tel: 800-776-7701/
408-438-1700
Fax: 408-438-7410

Simpler's Botanical
P.O. Box 2534
Sebastopol, CA 95473
Tel: 707-887-2012
Fax: 707-887-7570

Unitea Herbs
1705 14th Street
Suite 318
Boulder, CO 80302
Tel: 800-864-8327
(out of state)
Fax: 303-443-1248 (in state)

II. HERB SUPPLIERS—MAIL, PHONE, AND FAX ORDERS

The following companies sell **fresh plant herbs** and **seeds**.
Write, phone, or fax for product and ordering information.

Seeds of Change
P.O. Box 15700
Santa Fe, NM 87506-5700
Tel: 888-762-7333

Seed Savers Exchange
3076 North Winn Road
Decorah, IA 52101

Tel: 319-382-5990
Fax: 319-382-5872

Shepherd's Garden Seeds
30 Irene Street
Torrington, CT 06790
Tel: 860-482-3638
Fax: 860-482-0532

III. HERB SUPPLIERS—INTERNET

The following is a limited list of companies that sell herbs via their websites. Have a credit card handy.

BioSynergy Health
Alternatives
www.biosynergy.com, or
Tel: 800-554-7145
Fax: 208-342-0880

Reach4Life Quality Products
www.reach4life.com

Tenzing Momo, Inc.
www.tenzing.com, or
Tel: 800-365-9682
Fax: 206-728-4010

RESOURCES

American Holistic
Medical Association
6728 Old McLean
Village Drive
McLean, VA 22101
Tel: 703-556-9728
(To locate a holistic medical
practitioner)

American Association of
Naturopathic Physicians
601 Valley Street, Suite #105
Seattle, WA 98109
Tel: 206-298-0126
Fax: 206-298-0129
Referral Line: 206-298-0125
(To locate a naturopathic
physician)

ORGANIZATIONS

For the latest information about herbs and herbal medicine

American Botanical Council
P.O. Box 201660
Austin, TX 78720
Tel: 512-331-8868

American Herb Association
P.O. Box 1673
Nevada City, CA 95949
Tel: 916-265-9552

American Herbalists Guild
P.O. Box 746555
Arvada, CO 80006
Tel: 303-423-8800

Botanica Press
4680 Smith Grade
Santa Cruz, CA 95060
Tel: 408-457-9095
Fax: 408-457-9097

Herb Research Foundation
1007 Pearl Street
Suite 200
Boulder, CO 80302
Tel: 303-449-2265

The Herb Society of America
9019 Kirtland-Chardon Road
Kirtland, OH 44094
Tel: 216-256-0514

References

Chapter 1: The Story of St. John's Wort

Bloomfield, Harold H., and Peter McWilliams. *Hypericum & Depression* (Los Angeles: Prelude Press, 1996).

Buchman, Dian Dincin. *Herbal Medicine: The Natural Way to Get Well and Stay Well* (New York: Gramercy Publishing, 1980).

Duke, James A. *CRC Handbook of Medicinal Herbs* (Boca Raton, FL: CRC Press, 1985).

Heinerman, John. *Heinerman's Encyclopedia of Fruits, Vegetables and Herbs* (West Nyack, NY: Parker Publishing Company, 1988).

Hoffman, David. *The Complete Illustrated Holistic Herbal* (Rockport, MA: Element Books, 1996).

Lavie, G., et al. The chemical and biological properties of hypericin—compound with a broad spectrum of biological activities. *Medicinal Research Reviews* 15, no. 2(1995): 111–19.

Le Strange, Richard. *A History of Herbal Plants* (New York: Arco Publishing, 1977).

Linde, K., et al. St. John's wort for depression—an overview and meta-analysis of randomised clinical trials. *British Medical Journal* 313, no. 7052(1996): 253–58.

Lipp, Frank J. *Herbalism* (New York: Little, Brown, 1996).

Mills, Simon Y. *Out of the Earth: The Essential Book of Herbal Medicine* (New York: Viking, 1991).

Millspaugh, Charles F. *American Medicinal Plants* (New York: Dover Publications, 1974).

Mindell, Earl. *Earl Mindell's Herb Bible* (New York: Simon & Schuster, 1992).

Ody, Penelope. *The Complete Medicinal Herbal* (New York: Dorling Kindersley, 1993).

Pitman, Vicki. *Herbal Medicine: The Use of Herbs for Health and Healing* (Rockport, MA: Element Books, 1995).

Theiss, Barbara and Peter. *The Family Herbal: A Guide to Natural Health Care for Yourself and Your Children* (Rochester, VT: Healing Arts Press, 1989, 1993).

Zuess, Jonathan. *The Natural Prozac Program: How to Use St. John's Wort, the Antidepressant Herb* (New York: Three Rivers Press/Crown Publishers, 1997).

Chapter 2: The Magic of the Medicine

American Herbal Pharmacopoeia™ and Therapeutic Compendium. Monograph St. John's Wort, American Herbal Pharmacopoeia™, Santa Cruz, CA, 1997.

Berghöfer, R., and J. Hölzl. Biflavonoids in Hypericum perforatum, Part I. Isolation of 13, 118-biapigenin, *Planta Medica* (1987): 216–17.

Berghöfer, R., and J. Hölzl. Isolation of 13, 118-biapigenin (amentoflavone) from Hypericum perforatum, *Planta Medica* (1989): 91.

Bladt, S., and H. Wagner. Inhibition of MAO by fractions and constituents of Hypericum extract. *Journal of Geriatric Psychiatry and Neurology* 7 Suppl. 1(1994): S 57–59.

Brondz, I., T. Greibrokk, P. A. Groth, and A. J. Aasen. The Relative Stereochemistry of hyperforin—an antibiotic substance from Hypericum perforatum. *Tetrahedron Letters* 23(1982): 1299–1300.

Carpenter, S., and G. A. Kraus. Photosensitization is required for inactivation of equine infectious anemia virus by hypericin. *Photochemistry and Photobiology* 53(1991): 169–74.

Couldwell, W.T., R. Gopalakrishna, D.R. Hinton, et al. Hypericin: a potential antiglioma therapy. *Neurosurgery* 35(1994): 705–10.

Degar, S., G. Lavie, and D. Meruelo. Photodynamic inactivation of radiation leukemia virus produced from hypericin-treated cells. *Virology* 197(1993): 796–800.

Demisch, L., et al. Identification of MAO-type-A inhibitors in Hypericum perforatum L. (Hyperforat). *Pharmacopsychiatry* 22(1989): 194.

Duke, James A. *CRC Handbook of Medicinal Herbs* (Boca Raton, FL: CRC Press, 1985).

Ernst, E. St. John's wort, an anti-depressant? A systematic, criteria-based review. *Phytomedicine* 2(1995): 47–71.

Grinenko, N. A. The composition of flavonoids and derivatives of anthraquinone in Hypericum perforatum L. and H. maculatum. *Chemical Abstracts* 111(1989): 191523t.

Gurevich, A. I., V. N. Dobrynin, M. N. Kolosov, et al. Hyperforin, an antibiotic from Hypericum perforatum. *Antibiotiki* 16(1971): 510–13.

Hahn, G. Hypericum perforatum (St. John's wort)—a medicinal herb used in antiquity and still of interest today. *Journal of Naturopathic Medicine* 3(1992): 94–96.

Heinze, A., and H. Göbel. Hypericum perforans in the treatment of chronic tension-type headache. *2nd International Congress on Phytomedicine,* Munich, 1996.

Hobbs, C. St. John's wort: Hypericum perforatum L. A review. *HerbalGram* 18/19(1989): 24–33.

Hoffman, David. *The Complete Illustrated Holistic Herbal* (Rockport, MA: Element Books, 1996).

Hudson, J. B., I. Lopez-Bazzocchi, and G. H. Towers. Antiviral activities of hypericin. *Antiviral Research* 15(1991): 101–12.

Kartnig, T., I. Göbel, and B. Heydel. Production of hypericin, pseudohypericin and flavonoids in cell cultures of various Hypericum species and their chemotypes. *Planta Medica* 62(1996): 51–53.

Kerb, R., et al. Single-dose and steady-state pharmacokinetics of hypericin and pseudohypericin. *Antimicrobial Agents and Chemotherapy* 40(1996): 2087–93.

Khosa, R. L., and N. Bhatia. Antifungal effect of Hypericum perforatum. *Journal of Scientific Research and Plants Medicine* 3 (1982): 49–50.

Kook, A. I., et al. Depression and immunity: the biochemical interrelationship between the central nervous system and the immune system. *Biological Psychiatry* 37(1995): 817–19.

Lavie, G., et al. Hypericin as an inactivator of infectious viruses in blood components. *Transfusion* 35 (1995): 392–400.

Lavie, G., et al. Studies of the mechanisms of the antiretroviral agents hypericin and pseudohypericin. *Proceedings of the National Academy of Sciences of the United States of America* 86(1989): 5963–67.

Lavie, G., et al. The chemical and biological properties of hypericin—compound with a broad spectrum of biological activities. *Medicinal Research Reviews* 15(1995): 111–19.

Le Strange, Richard. *A History of Herbal Plants* (New York: Arco Publishing, 1977).

Linde, K., et al. St. John's wort for depression—an overview and meta-analysis of randomised clinical trials. *British Medical Journal* 313, no. 7052(1996): 253–58.

Melzer, R., U. Fricke, and J. Hölzl. Vasoactive properties of proanthocyanidins from Hypericum perforatum L. in isolated porcine coronary arteries. *Arzneimittel-Forschung* 41(1991): 481–83.

Meruelo, D., G. Lavie, and D. Lavie. Therapeutic agents with dramatic antiretroviral activity and little toxicity at effective doses: aromatic polycyclic diones hypericin and pseudohypericin. *Proceedings of the National Academy of Sciences of the United States of America* 85(1988): 5230–34.

Mills, Simon Y. *Out of the Earth: The Essential Book of Herbal Medicine* (New York: Viking, 1991).

Millspaugh, Charles F. *American Medicinal Plants* (New York: Dover Publications, 1974).

Muller, W. E., et al., Effects of Hypericum extract LI 160 on neurotransmitter uptake systems and adrenergic receptor density. *2nd International Congress on Phytomedicine*, Munich, 1996.

Muller, W. E., and R. Rossol. Effects of Hypericum extract on the suppression of serotonin receptors. *Journal of Geriatric Psychiatry and Neurology* 7 Suppl. 1(1994): S63–64.

Nahrstedt, A., and V. Butterweck. Biologically active and other chemical constituents of the herb of Hypericum perforatum L. *Pharmacopsychiatry*, 1997 (in press).

Panossian, A. G., et al. Immunosuppressive effects of hypericin on stimulated human leucocytes: inhibition of the arachidonic acid release, leukotriene B4 and interleukin-1 production and activation of nitric oxide formation. *Phytomedicine* 3(1996): 19–28.

Rao, S. G., et al. Calendula and Hypericum: two homeopathic drugs promoting wound healing in rats. *Fitoterapia* 6(1991): 508–10.

Shipochliev, T. Extracts from a group of medicinal plants enhancing uterine tonus. *Veterinarno-Meditenski Nauki* 18(1981): 87–94.

Sommer, H., and G. Harrer. Placebo-controlled double-blind study examining the effectiveness of a Hypericum preparation in 105 mildly depressed patients. *Journal of Geriatric Psychiatry and Neurology* 7 Suppl. 1(1994): S 9–11.

Steinbeck, K. A., and P. Wernet. Successful long-term treatment over 40 months of HIV-patients with intravenous hypericin. *International Conference on AIDS*. Germany; 1993; Abstract #PO-B26-2012.

Stevenson, N. R., and J. Lenard. Antiretroviral activities of hypericin and rose bengal: photodynamic effects on Friend leukemia virus infection of mice. *Antiviral Research* 21(1993): 119–27.

Suzuki, O., et al. Inhibition of monoamine oxidase by hypericin. *Planta Medica* 50(1984): 272–74.

Takahashi, I., et al. Hypericin and pseudohypericin specifically inhibit protein kinase C; possible relation to their anti-retroviral activity. *Biochemical and Biophysical Research Committee* 165 (1989): 1207–12.

Theiss, Barbara and Peter. *The Family Herbal: A Guide to Natural Health Care for Yourself and Your Children* (Rochester, VT: Healing Arts Press, 1989, 1993).

Vickery, A. R. Traditional uses and folklore of hypericum in the British Isles. *Economic Botany* (1981): 289–95.

Weber, N. D., et al. The antiviral agent hypericin has in vitro activity against HSV-1 through nonspecific association with viral and cellular membranes. *Antiviral Chemistry & Chemotherapy* 5 (1994): 83–90.

Wölk, H., G. Burkard, and J. Grunwald. Benefits and risks of the hypericum extract LI 160: drug monitoring study with 3250 patients. *Journal of Geriatric Psychiatry and Neurology* 7 Suppl. 1(1994): S 34–38.

Wood, S., et al. Antiviral activity of naturally occurring anthraquinones and anthraquinone derivatives. *Planta Medica* 56 (1990): 651–652.

Yip, L., et al. Antiviral activity of a derivative of the photosensitive compound hypericin. *Phytomedicine* 3 (1996): 185–90.

Zuess, Jonathan. *The Natural Prozac Program: How to Use St. John's Wort, the Antidepressant Herb* (New York: Three Rivers Press/Crown Publishers, 1997).

Chapter 3: Is St. John's Wort for Everyone?

American Herbal Pharmacopoeia™ and Therapeutic Compendium. Monograph St. John's Wort, American Herbal Pharmacopoeia™, Santa Cruz, CA, 1997.

Linde, K., et al. St. John's wort for depression—an overview and meta-analysis of randomised clinical trials. *British Medical Journal* 313, no. 7052(1996): 253–58.

Mills, Simon Y. *Out of the Earth: The Essential Book of Herbal Medicine* (New York: Viking, 1991).

Sommer, H., and G. Harrer. Placebo-controlled double-blind study examining the effectiveness of a Hypericum preparation in 105 mildly depressed patients. *Journal of Geriatric Psychiatry and Neurology* 7 Suppl. 1(1994): S 9–11.

Wölk, H., G. Burkard, and J. Grunwald. Benefits and risks of the Hypericum extract LI 160: drug monitoring study with 3250 patients. *Journal of Geriatric Psychiatry and Neurology* 7 Suppl. 1 (1994): S 34–38.

Zuess, Jonathan. *The Natural Prozac Program: How to Use St. John's Wort, the Antidepressant Herb* (New York: Three Rivers Press/Crown Publishers, 1997).

Chapter 4: Finding St. John's Wort

Hoffman, David. *The Complete Illustrated Holistic Herbal* (Rockport, MA: Element Books, 1996).

Mills, Simon Y. *Out of the Earth: The Essential Book of Herbal Medicine* (New York: Viking, 1991).

Chapter 5: Treating Depression with St. John's Wort

American Herbal Pharmacopoeia™ and Therapeutic Compendium. Monograph St. John's Wort, American Herbal Pharmacopoeia™, Santa Cruz, CA, 1997.

Bladt, S., and H. Wagner. Inhibition of MAO by fractions and constituents of Hypericum extract. *Journal of Geriatric Psychiatry and Neurology* 7 Suppl. 1(1994): S 57–59.

Bloomfield, Harold H., and Peter McWilliams. *Hypericum & Depression* (Los Angeles: Prelude Press, 1996).

Demisch, L., et al. Identification of MAO-type-A inhibitors in Hypericum perforatum L. (Hyperforat). *Pharmacopsychiatry* 22 (1989): 194.

Duke, James A. *CRC Handbook of Medicinal Herbs* (Boca Raton, FL: CRC Press, 1985).

Ernst, E. St. John's wort, an anti-depressant? A systematic, criteria-based review. *Phytomedicine* 2 (1995): 47–71.

Hobbs, C. St. John's wort: Hypericum perforatum L. A review. *HerbalGram* 18/19 (1989): 24–33.

Kook, A. I., et al. Depression and immunity: the biochemical interrelationship between the central nervous system and the immune system. *Biological Psychiatry* 37 (1995): 817–19.

Lavie, G., et al. The chemical and biological properties of hypericin—compound with a broad spectrum of biological activities. *Medicinal Research Reviews* 15, no. 2(1995): 111–19.

Linde, K., et al. St. John's wort for depression—an overview and meta-analysis of randomised clinical trials. *British Medical Journal* 313, no. 7052(1996): 253–58.

Muller, W. E., et al. Effects of Hypericum extract LI 160 on neurotransmitter uptake systems and adrenergic receptor density. *2nd International Congress on Phytomedicine,* Munich, 1996.

Muller, W. E., and R. Rossol. Effects of Hypericum extract on the suppression of serotonin receptors. *Journal of Geriatric Psychiatry and Neurology* 7 Suppl. 1 (1994): S63–64.

Nahrstedt, A., and V. Butterweck. Biologically active and other chemical constituents of the herb of Hypericum perforatum L. *Pharmacopsychiatry,* 1997 (in press).

The New Good Housekeeping *Family Health and Medical Guide* (New York: William Morrow, 1989).

Panossian, A. G., et al. Immunosuppressive effects of hypericin on stimulated human leucocytes: inhibition of the arachidonic acid release, leukotriene B4 and interleukin-1 production and activation of nitric oxide formation. *Phytomedicine* 3(1996): 19–28.

Sommer, H., and G. Harrer. Placebo-controlled double-blind

study examining the effectiveness of a Hypericum preparation in 105 mildly depressed patients. *Journal of Geriatric Psychiatry and Neurology* 7 Suppl. 1(1994) S 9–11.

Suzuki, O., et al. Inhibition of monoamine oxidase by hypericin. *Planta Medica* 50(1984): 272–74.

Theiss, Barbara and Peter. *The Family Herbal: A Guide to Natural Health Care for Yourself and Your Children* (Rochester, VT: Healing Arts Press, 1989, 1993).

Vickery, A. R. Traditional uses and folklore of hypericum in the British Isles. *Economic Botany* (1981): 289–95.

Wölk, H., G. Burkard, and J. Grunwald. Benefits and risks of the hypericum extract LI 160: drug monitoring study with 3250 patients. *Journal of Geriatric Psychiatry and Neurology* 7 Suppl. 1(1994): S 34–38.

Zuess, Jonathan. *The Natural Prozac Program: How to Use St. John's Wort, the Antidepressant Herb* (New York: Three Rivers Press/Crown Publishers, 1997).

Chapter 6: Treating PMS, Menstrual Problems, and Menopausal Symptoms

American Herbal Pharmacopoeia™ and Therapeutic Compendium. Monograph St. John's Wort, American Herbal Pharmacopoeia™, Santa Cruz, CA, 1997.

Hahn, G. Hypericum perforatum (St. John's wort)—a medicinal herb used in antiquity and still of interest today. *Journal of Naturopathic Medicine* 3(1992): 94–96.

Heinze, A., and H. Göbel. Hypericum perforans in the treatment of chronic tension-type headache. *2nd International Congress on Phytomedicine,* Munich, 1996.

Hobbs, C. St. John's wort: Hypericum perforatum L. A review. *HerbalGram* 18/19(1989): 24–33.

Hoffman, David. *The Complete Illustrated Holistic Herbal* (Rockport, MA: Element Books, 1996).

Lavie, G., et al. The chemical and biological properties of hypericin—compound with a broad spectrum of biological activities. *Medicinal Research Reviews* 15, no. 2(1995): 111–19.

Linde, K., et al. St. John's wort for depression—an overview and meta-analysis of randomised clinical trials. *British Medical Journal* 313, no. 7052(1996): 253–58.

Mills, Simon Y. *Out of the Earth: The Essential Book of Herbal Medicine* (New York: Viking, 1991).

Millspaugh, Charles F. *American Medicinal Plants* (New York: Dover Publications, 1974).

Panossian, A. G., et al. Immunosuppressive effects of hypericin on stimulated human leucocytes: inhibition of the arachidonic acid release, leukotriene B4 and interleukin-1 production and activation of nitric oxide formation. *Phytomedicine* 3(1996): 19–28.

Pitman, Vicki. *Herbal Medicine: The Use of Herbs for Health and Healing* (Rockport, MA: Element Books, 1995).

Shipochliev, T. Extracts from a group of medicinal plants enhancing uterine tonus. *Veterinarno-Meditenski Nauki* 18(1981): 87–94.

Theiss, Barbara and Peter. *The Family Herbal: A Guide to Natural Health Care for Yourself and Your Children* (Rochester, VT: Healing Arts Press, 1989, 1993).

Zuess, Jonathan. *The Natural Prozac Program: How to Use St. John's Wort, the Antidepressant Herb* (New York: Three Rivers Press/Crown Publishers, 1997).

Chapter 7: Treating Insomnia with St. John's Wort

Johnson, D., et al. Effects of hypericum extract LI 160 compared with maprotiline on resting EEG and evoked potentials in 24 volunteers. *Journal of Geriatric Psychiatry and Neurology* 7 Suppl. 1(1994): S 44–46.

The New Good Housekeeping *Family Health and Medical Guide* (New York: William Morrow, 1989).

Schultz, H. and M. Jobert. Effects of hypericum extract on the sleep EEG in older volunteers. *Journal of Geriatric Psychiatry and Neurology* 7 Suppl. 1(1994): S 39–43.

Chapter 8: Fighting Viruses and Strengthening Immunity with St. John's Wort

American Herbal Pharmacopoeia™ and Therapeutic Compendium. Monograph St. John's Wort, American Herbal Pharmacopoeia™, Santa Cruz, CA, 1997.

Hobbs, C. St. John's wort: Hypericum perforatum L. A review. *HerbalGram* 18/19 (1989): 24–33.

Hoffman, David. *The Complete Illustrated Holistic Herbal* (Rockport, MA: Element Books, 1996).

Hudson, J. B., I. Lopez-Bazzocchi, and G. H. Towers. Antiviral activities of hypericin. *Antiviral Research* 15 (1991): 101–12.

Kook, A. I., et al. Depression and immunity: the biochemical interrelationship between the central nervous system and the immune system. *Biological Psychiatry* 37 (1995): 817–19.

Lavie, G., et al. The chemical and biological properties of hypericin—compound with a broad spectrum of biological activities. *Medicinal Research Reviews* 15(1995): 111–19.

Lavie, G., et al. Hypericin as an inactivator of infectious viruses in blood components. *Transfusion* 35 (1995): 392–400.

Lavie, G., et al. Studies of the mechanisms of the antiretroviral agents hypericin and pseudohypericin. *Proceedings of the National Academy of Sciences of the United States of America* 86(1989): 5963–67.

Meruelo, D., G. Lavie, and D. Lavie. Therapeutic agents with dramatic antiretroviral activity and little toxicity at effective doses: aromatic polycyclic diones hypericin and pseudohypericin. *Proceedings of the National Academy of Sciences of the United States of America* 85 (1988): 5230–34.

Nahrstedt, A., and V. Butterweck. Biologically active and other chemical constituents of the herb of Hypericum perforatum L. *Pharmacopsychiatry,* 1997 (in press).

The New Good Housekeeping *Family Health and Medical Guide* (New York: William Morrow, 1989).

Panossian, A. G., et al. Immunosuppressive effects of hypericin on stimulated human leucocytes: inhibition of the arachidonic acid release, leukotriene B4 and interleukin-1 production and activation of nitric oxide formation. *Phytomedicine* 3(1996): 19–28.

Stevenson, N. R., and J. Lenard. Antiretroviral activities of hypericin and rose bengal: photodynamic effects on Friend leukemia virus infection of mice. *Antiviral Research* 21 (1993): 119–27.

Weber, N. D., et al. The antiviral agent hypericin has in vitro activity against HSV-1 through nonspecific association with viral and cellular membranes. *Antiviral Chemistry & Chemotherapy* 5(1994): 83–90.

Wood, S., et al. Antiviral activity of naturally occurring anthraquinones and anthraquinone derivatives. *Planta Medica* 56 (1990): 651–52.

Yip, L., et al. Antiviral activity of a derivative of the photosensitive compound hypericin. *Phytomedicine* 3 (1996): 185–90.

Zuess, Jonathan. *The Natural Prozac Program: How to Use St. John's Wort, the Antidepressant Herb* (New York: Three Rivers Press/Crown Publishers, 1997).

Chapter 9: Achieving Weight Loss with St. John's Wort

Personal Communication with Steven Blechman, Twin Laboratories, and Dr. David Allison, New York Obesity Research Center, November 1997.

Chapter 10: Looking Ahead

American Herbal Pharmacopoeia™ and Therapeutic Compendium. Monograph St. John's Wort, American Herbal Pharmacopoeia™, Santa Cruz, CA, 1997.

Couldwell, W.T., R. Gopalakrishna, D.R. Hinton, et al. Hypericin: a potential antiglioma therapy. *Neurosurgery* 35 (1994): 705–10.

Heinze, A., and H. Göbel. Hypericum perforans in the treatment of chronic tension-type headache. *2nd International Congress on Phytomedicine,* Munich, 1996.

Lavie, G., et al. Hypericin as an inactivator of infectious viruses in blood components. *Transfusion* 35(1995): 392–400.

Melzer, R., U. Fricke, and J. Hölzl. Vasoactive properties of proanthocyanidins from Hypericum perforatum L. in isolated porcine coronary arteries. *Arzneimittel-Forschung* 41(1991): 481–83.

Nahrstedt, A., and V. Butterweck. Biologically active and other chemical constituents of the herb of Hypericum perforatum L. *Pharmacopsychiatry,* 1997 (in press).

Index